DISCLAIMER

While anyone may find the exercises and ideas in this book to be useful, it is sold with the understanding that the author is not engaged in presenting specific psychological advice. Nor is anything in this book intended to be a diagnosis, prescription, recommendation, or cure for any specific kind of medical or psychological problem. Each person has unique needs, and this book cannot take these individual differences into account. So, while this book can feel relatable and accurate and, in many cases, cause extremely profound shifts in cognition, use your own judgment or that of a professional before making any significant life changes. The contents in this book only apply to individuals who have their basic physical needs met as the nature of this information is irrelevant until that point.

ENLIGHTENED ENOUGH

A SELF MASTERY BOOK TO STOP OVERTHINKING, ESCAPE SELF SABOTAGE, AND IMPROVE YOUR MIND AND EMOTIONS

JUSTIN QUINTON

WWW.ACTUALIZE.ACADEMY

HOW TO READ THIS BOOK

This is unlike most books you will commonly come across that are slower-paced and filled with fluff to explain a few simple points. Instead, this book is condensed and its writing is heavy at times. You might find yourself wanting to put this book down to process what you just read or even give up trying to understand what is being presented, this is perfectly okay. If you find yourself lost with a concept, just continue reading past it. The ideas from prior pages tend to become clearer as you read on. You might find yourself well into this book and still confused as to the point of it, again, this is expected.

Despite the fact that you might not have a specific goal when reading this book, it has a specific goal for you. To help you reach a temporary state of enlightenment that simplifies your thoughts and life.

In aiming at this goal, there are 3 different types of reader experiences that typically happen:

> **1)** The ideas start to build on each other, and you get small progressive insights that collectively add up to a profound understanding by the end.
>
> **2)** You find yourself lost with the ideas, not understanding how they relate to you or what points the book is trying to make. Perhaps you find the content repetitive until suddenly something clicks and you're struck with a profound clarity.
>
> **3)** While reading this you become irritable because it seems like nonsensical psycho-babble that is just trying to sound profound. If this is the case, try reading this at another point in your life.

But regardless of your degree of comprehension, you can get the most out of this book by taking the time to actually think through the exercises and questions presented. While you might learn new things, emotionally understanding these ideas is much more important than just cognitively knowing them.

Lastly, this book has been broken down into 3 parts, which all have different styles of writing in them. Each one becomes easier and more enjoyable as you progress through the book.

Part 1 is Psychology.

Part 2 is Philosophy.

Part 3 is Personal Development.

In other words, the "who & what", the "when & why", and the "how".

CONTENTS

PART I
MIND & BODY

PART II
LIFE & BEING

PART III
LIVING & ACTION

PART I
MIND & BODY

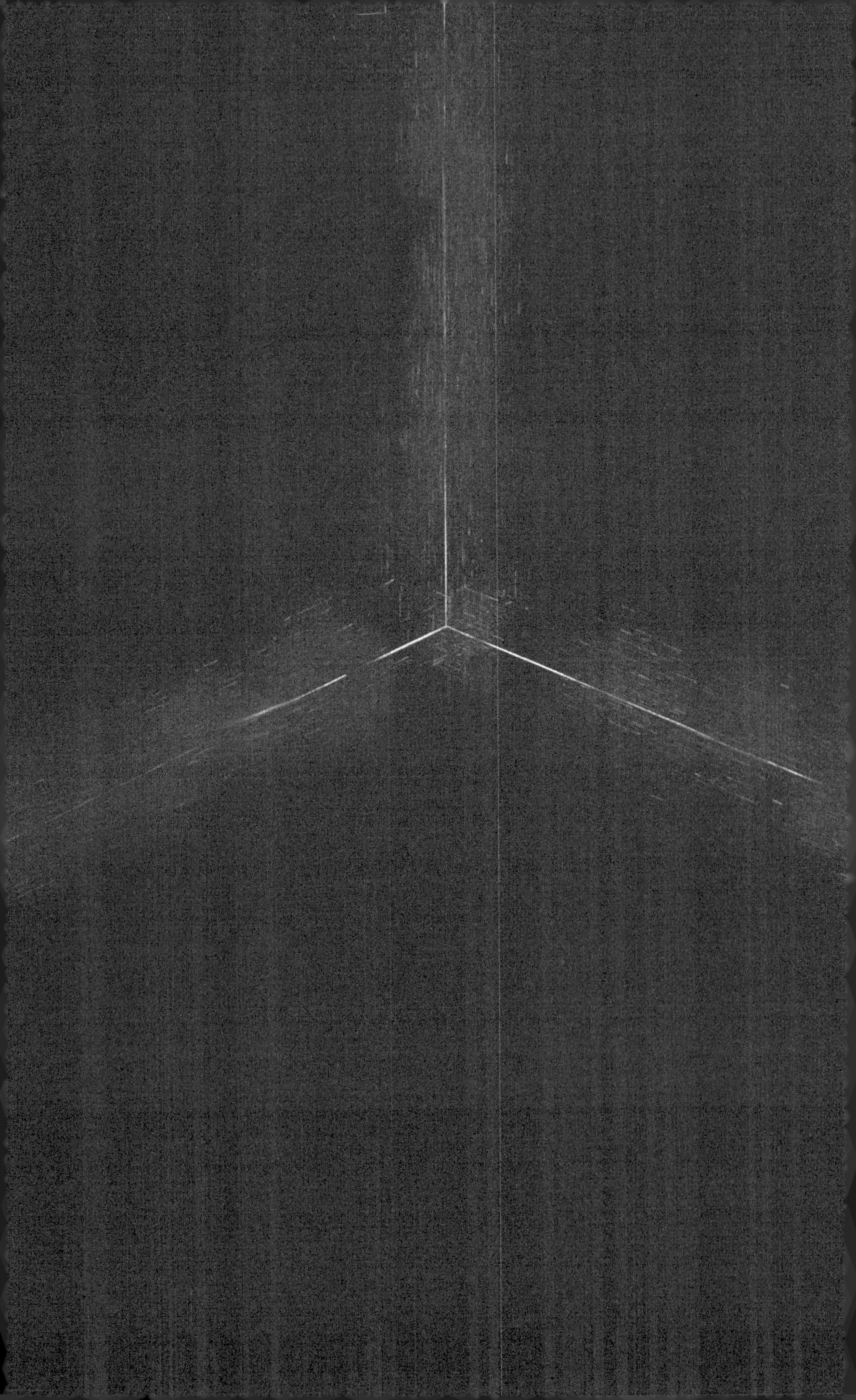

CHAPTER ONE

WHY THIS BOOK IS FOR YOU

| THE DARK ROOM |

Imagine being placed in a dark room, unable to see anything around you. As you try to feel your way around the room, you first make contact with a wall. Keeping your hand on the wall, you slowly guide yourself into the corner of the room. Once there, you take a moment to orient yourself and decide to explore further, again blindly hugging the new wall as you move across the room. Before you can reach the end, you're startled by your foot getting tangled with something on the ground. You frantically flail your foot around, shaking the lengthy mass off you as you dart back to the other side of the room. Now back in your corner, your imagination races with possibilities as you try to make out what that was. While you try to calm down and use your logic to help you determine the many things it could have been. You can't help but feel a sense of unease as your mind solidifies the idea that you're sharing this room with a snake curled up in the other corner.

As a precautionary measure, you have decided that you should stay away from that corner, but the rest of the room should be fine. Yet, despite following this rule, you still find yourself thinking of the snake. You worry that its location has changed or that you're too close to it as you move around the room. As time passes, this worrying grows into stress and hatred for the snake. Eventually, you begin fantasizing about how much better your experience would be if the snake didn't exist or how much easier your life would be if you could just kill it. While pacing around in the comfortable parts of the room, this collection of thoughts builds up into a desire that has you consumed in your mind. Lost in your imagination of living without the snake, you picture yourself dancing in the room, running around, and being carefree. You suddenly realize you no longer know where you are in the room as this is happening.

Frantically you spin around, searching for something to orient yourself to; in this panic, you think you hear the snake move. Immediately, you freeze where you are, stiffen your posture, and silence your breath. As you try to listen, you can only make out your heartbeat and stifled breathing. This only infuriates you more as you decide to make a desperate lunge towards any corner. As you bolt into an unknown direction, you're once again met by a wall. With your last burst of bravery, you charge towards a corner, and luckily it happens to be a safe one.

Curled up in a ball and riddled in fear, you cope with this experience by creating even more rules to ensure this never happens again. Forget about pacing or moving about; you now need to stay put in your corner. You also decide to keep your focus on your surroundings, not letting your imagination wander off as it did before. Armed with these and a few more limitations, you think you should be able to keep safe as long as you remain committed to following them. However, your experience is still one of feeling unsafe regardless of your efforts.

So as you sit still and quiet in the corner of the room, a slight hum starts to hiss above you. It is the sound of fluorescent light bulbs beginning to illuminate.

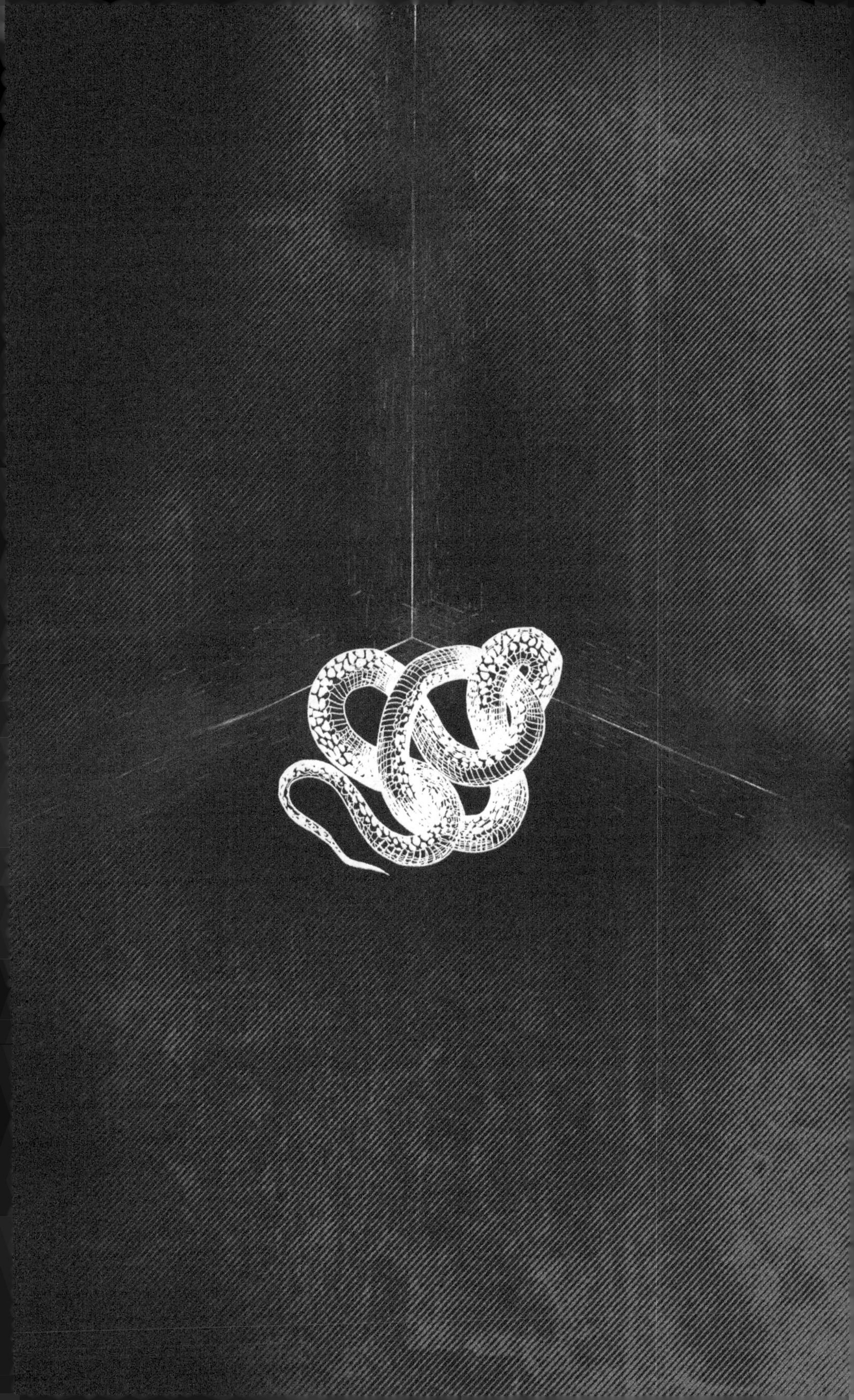

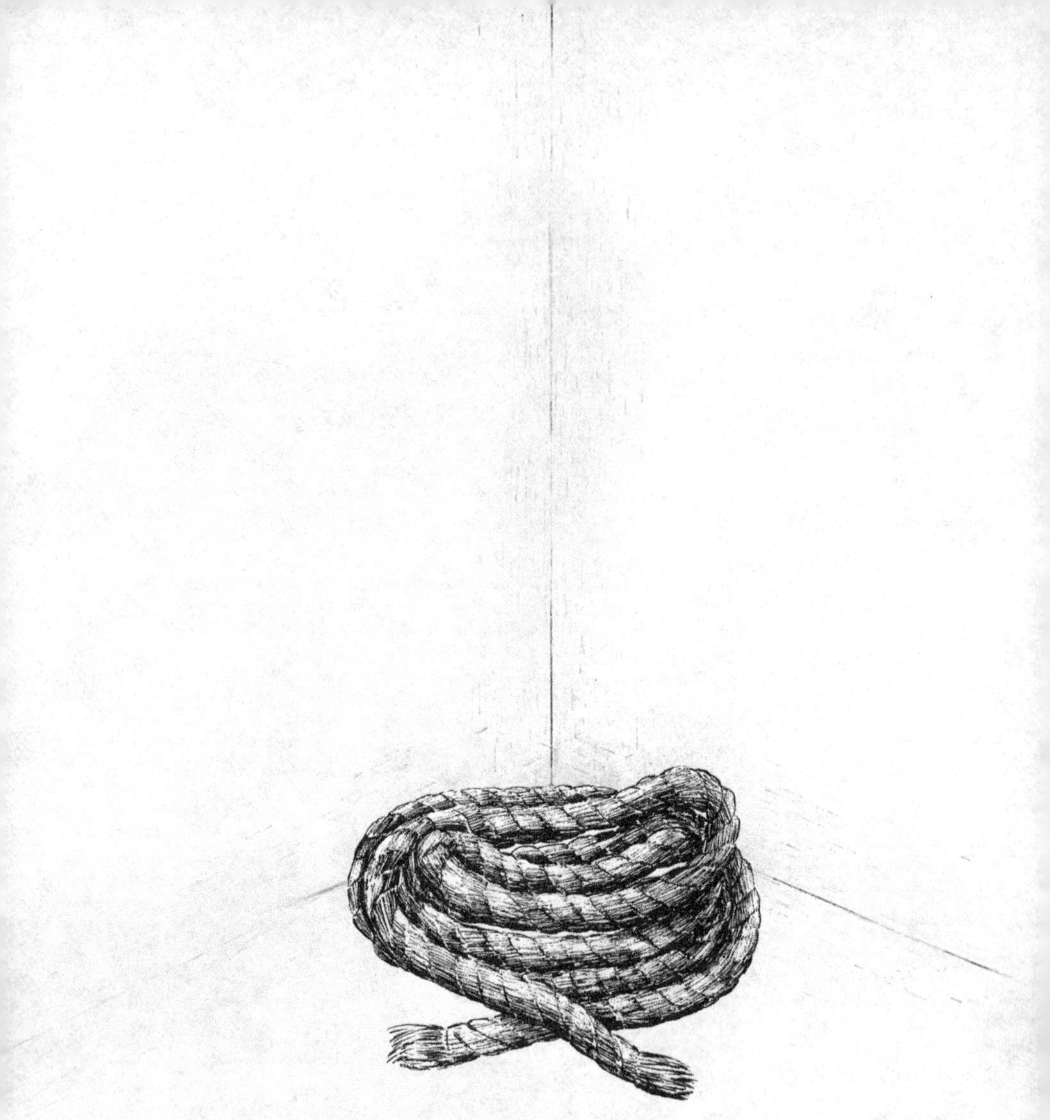

Suddenly, they burst into full brightness, blinding you as they light up the entire room. As your eyes adjust, you squint your attention to each of the corners, fearfully watching as your vision regains focus and this curled-up snake starts to materialize. You stare in absolute horror as you try to make out the details of the snake. However, as your view sharpens, you become aware that this curled-up figure is not a snake. Instead, it is just a bundle of rolled-up rope. You approach the corner of the room and pick it up in relief and surprise as you confirm that it has just been a rope all this time. After a few more moments, the lights then turn back off.

Again, you find yourself in this dark room, only this time, it is entirely different. There is no more fear and no more anger. The rules that you once held tightly to no longer serve you. You feel a wave of ease and enjoyment wash over you as this newfound freedom emerges. So, as you stand in this same darkroom, though nothing has actually changed about it, it feels completely different.

This is the experience I hope to give you with this book. I want to help you shine a light on the areas of your mind that most people are frightened to delve into. In this, you will experience a newfound sense of possibility and freedom that had previously been hidden in the dark. You will not find anything in this book that changes the content of your life but rather the context. When you do this, the way you show up in your current circumstances will change, along with many decisions that used to make sense. You will experience a new range of emotions once lost. You will also find freedom from the very things that once silently held you back in life.

My role in this is not to be smarter than you or be some guru who is immune to the topics of this book. Instead, I am just an observer of my own life and inviting you to look at these human qualities we all share. I'm not asking you to believe in any religion or idea, and I'm not even asking you to trust what I'm saying. Rather, see this as an invitation to turn a light on in your own darkroom and inquire alongside me into the snakes of your own life.

| WHAT YOU CAN EXPECT FROM THIS |

While I do not know who you are or where you are in your life when reading this, I do know a few things that are universal to the experience of life.

Human beings have problems and struggles.

Maybe it is a job that drains you. Maybe it is a relationship that you are uncertain about. Maybe it is a memory from your past that keeps haunting you. Maybe it is a negative circumstance or environment that you want to get away from. Maybe it is an emotion like jealousy or anger or fear that continually obsesses your mind. Maybe it is an addiction or compulsive behavior you are hiding from others.

While this might feel like an impossible statement to believe as you start reading this book now, the job, relationship, memory, or situation that once drained you, could also become the very thing that inspires and revitalizes you. This isn't about positive thinking or doing something anti-intellectual in which you pretend life is not the way it is, or purposefully ignoring something. It is about using a philosophy to clarify how your life shows up for you and the way you show up within it. In which you can observe the *being* part of what makes you a human being. How the things we call "you" or "I" show up in our heads as the thoughts that make up our experience.

See, as you come to understand this philosophy, you will be able to remove the complications and confusions you may have around your life. This philosophy tends to simplify our lives so that we can see even lifelong issues with a clarity that provides freedom from them. Be it financial issues, relationship complications, troubled pasts, or insecurities. When a person is no longer held down by these very human challenges, they tend to show up with more motivation, more happiness, and more purpose in life. What shows up is a childlike excitement, a deep desire to engage and sink your teeth into what you do and to make a difference, alongside contentment about your life, that regardless of the outcome, you will be just fine. Again, this does not come from some illogical or faith-oriented idea. But from one that is grounded in a very pragmatic, observable philosophy that you can immediately experience and test for yourself. Because of this, I do not have to ask you to suspend your critical thinking or to believe anything I believe. Rather, all you need to do is just observe and think for yourself on how the different ideas in this book apply to your life and those around you.

It is a safe assumption to make that you are currently skeptical about the claims of experiencing a better life, and rightly so. Again, this is not about pretending the challenges of your life do not currently exist and are not real. Your disbelief about any book changing those circumstances is logical.

The numbers in your bank account are very real, the time you spend arguing or fighting with people is real, the effort you apply trying to stop incessant insecure thoughts is real, the unreliable car, or ending of a relationship is real. Those things matter and this book is not here to convince you otherwise. Rather, this book is an invitation to observe in what way they matter and show up so that you can see them for what they actually are, and not as they feel. See, the amount of money you do or do not have is real, but what you believe and feel about it is not, it is subjective. Our feelings come from an intangible series of thoughts that collectively make up an assessment about what that amount of money means. This then has us fearful or excited for the future and what comes. But it is anti-intellectual to assume that all it takes is reframing those real issues or that painting over them with positivity is enough to solve them. In order to logically gain lasting clarity and improvement to the experience of your life that this book claims, we need to look at why we have these meanings in the first place and the depth at which they show up in all areas of life.

You would likely agree that if you could only solve a few or many pesky issues in your life, things would be perfect. Be it your fitness, relationships, or finances. That if these things were perfect by your standards, the quality of your life would improve. Or that if you could only figure out your purpose, you would feel happy and have endless motivation. Well, it is these beliefs that are at the very root of why motivation, happiness, and purpose seem to be hard to maintain and keep. In that, trying to find your purpose is almost a perfect way to never have one. Trying to be happy with forced positivity is almost a guaranteed way to never truly experience it. Trying to willpower your way into consistent motivation will only ever make you need more willpower. This is because these emotional states of motivation, happiness, and purpose are better had as reactions that show up, rather than forced objectives to be achieved.

This book will not dive into how to solve these issues with more productivity, positivity, and passion. Rather, it will help point out the nature of our need for these, so we can make way for those states to show up naturally and effortlessly. This is done with a philosophy that is built on the knowledge we gain through observation about what we are, who we are, and how we are when it comes to our lives.

So, just as with the example of the imagined snake, when we try to improve our finances, fitness, relationships, or any other area in life, we often fail to address the underlying motive that creates those ambitions. This activates our tendency to blindly apply more effort into how we behave, more pressure to control what we feel, and more exhaustive overthinking as an attempt to solve our current circumstances. Never addressing the issue of the snake itself, only temporarily suppressing the imagined fear of our encounter with it.

Like the rules to avoid the snake, we create rules of achievement to avoid the fact that we have to DO something in order to experience motivation, happiness, and purpose. It is the endless effort to ignore the "snake" that we are not naturally happy and content by default and that our happiness and contentment are only found through certain achievements or acknowledgments - all of which only let us temporarily feel safe from this snake. So, we make ourselves busy with the never-ending acquisition of them.

This also causes us to interpret those achievements as happiness when they are really just the temporary absence of fearful imagined outcomes. This is also why they never last, because our imaginations are very good at creating endless possibilities for things to go wrong, giving us endless hurdles to get over. Be it the need for a new job, promotion, business, relationship, experience, toy, vacation, achievement, or accolade.

Again, I'm not suggesting these things do not matter and make a difference to someone's experience. Instead, I'm suggesting that they do not get to the heart of the issue, which is our obsessive need for them in order to not be unhappy. This is how our lives are often composed of ways to avoid the snake, rather than facing it.

This book will dive into why this happens and how to face the snakes of our lives in more depth later. But first, it is important to understand what we are truly after, which is freedom from our snake. A lasting solution to motivation, happiness, and purpose. Not just more rules or things to achieve and do in an attempt to get those emotional states. This is why we need to identify and shine a light on this so-called snake in order for us to actually get what we are after.

When we do this, it does not feel like an achievement, but rather a relief - like looking at your bank statement after weeks of careless spending, only to find out you had more money than you anticipated, or a clean bill of health after a checkup you hesitated to get. It is a relief from the mental imagery that drives our compulsive actions to avoid fears. A freedom from the need to protect our insecurities, all of which creates a space for real motivation, happiness, and purpose to show up.

Just like our example, in the beginning, the snake is not something we can directly point out with our senses. We cannot see it with our eyes or feel it with our hands, yet it still remains very real as an experience. The way we experience the snake is through other means. We experience this snake through the fearful images of it in our minds, through the ideas we have around avoiding it, and through the wishes, we have for a life without it. The snake only exists through the reaction of thinking. It is the act of thinking that makes it possible for the snake to show up. It is that 'act' that makes it a real thing to avoid. So, without thinking fearful and dissatisfying thoughts, our snake cannot exist. Our challenge now is having to use our thinking to find a snake that only exists through our thinking - which is a lot like trying to taste your own tongue.

Now, unlike our example of the dark room, most of us are not aware of the snake. Instead, we only experience the consequences that come from living with the snake. This is because those ambitions and desires are very valid to us. The more we invest into them, the more we experience them as valid, never questioning why they exist in the first place. Moving away from our analogy, this looks like:

- Earning more money to avoid stressing about it
- Needing more passion in our relationships so we are less attracted to others
- Being more productive so we can stop beating ourselves up for a lack of results
- Achieving more success as a way of proving to ourselves and others that we are not failures

These may seem logical - and to some degree, they are. But they are ultimately ineffective as solutions to the origins of why these ambitions exist in the first place, which can be found by questioning:

Why are we not happy by default?

Why are we not productive by default?

Why are we never satisfied?

Our goal is not to answer those questions right now. But rather, to observe how the mechanisms that contain our inherent dissatisfaction function in our lives. Understanding these mechanisms lets us shine a light on the snake that validates those efforts to begin with - like, realizing it is a rope so we no longer need to manage it.

CHAPTER TWO

WHAT IS & WHAT IS NOT

| THE CONTENT OF LIFE |

Returning to our example of the snake, what changed when the lights turned on and it was revealed to just be a rope? Everything yet nothing. Nothing in the sense that the content of the room and the physical objects all remained the same. But everything in the sense that our thoughts toward the content changed.

It is the thoughts we have toward the content in our life that creates our experience.

Without them, the content remains meaningless, and having an experience of that content cannot exist. Think about the way in which your thoughts show up as an opinion on the thing you are focused on. Until you do this, you cannot experience that thing. Think of the many T-shirts you no longer wear, sitting in your dresser at home. Until you thought about them and remembered which of them you still had memories, opinions, or assessments on, they did not exist as an experience to you. Rather, they existed without meaning, just as they are - fabric in the shape of a torso, folded away. It is through the process of thinking that we decide what is important, good, bad, or stylish.

Your life and the contents within it are no different. Everything exists just as it is. Your job, relationships, and life. But it is our thought that lets us experience that content through the meanings that come with our thought.

Your life exists without meaning until you experience the thought that attaches meaning to it. The reason this may be difficult to grasp at first is that experience cannot exist without meaning, and vice versa. This is what makes the distinction of what is content versus meaning difficult to separate. This is why we cheer for sports teams we are not involved with, get angry at stories we hear on the news, and feel excited about hearing the latest work gossip. None of these things have anything to do with the content of our lives, yet we often make experiencing these meanings a huge part of our life.

This connection between meaning and content happens so automatically that we also forget that our thoughts are subjective and open to interpretation, which causes us to feel like we are accurately and objectively placing meaning to the content of our lives.

We think:

- "It must be a bad thing that I did not get the promotion I wanted"
- "Going through a breakup is the worst thing that could happen to me"
- "Having an unreliable car is embarrassing"

While all of those thoughts might feel accurate, they are still just subjective meanings we place to objective content. Even if we change the meanings to the ones below:

- "That promotion might have caused me more stress and headache than it was worth"
- "That relationship needed to end for me to find the one I should have been with"
- "But having a fully paid-off car is cooler"

These thoughts are still just subjective meanings that are separate from the content of our lives.

This business of our thoughts attaching meaning to content happens so automatically that we rarely question it. The result of that then becomes a new content for our lives, in which we spend our time just managing the thoughts and meanings we are attached to.

The funny thing about our attachment to these thoughts and meanings is that we rarely pick them ourselves. They are, for the most part, a collection of different influences you did not choose, such as biological drives for food and sex, egotistical fantasies of your importance to others, as well as societal conditioning of what is been advertised and taught to you. If you truly examine your thoughts, how many of them are uniquely yours? How much of your time is wasted on defending meanings you did not decide? How many of your meanings did you consciously choose?

Until we recognize that we live in content yet perceive in thought, we are trapped in meanings that are not truly ours.

| WE DO NOT HAVE THOUGHTS, THOUGHTS HAVE US. |

In addition to our thoughts automatically attaching meaning to the content in our lives, we also have very little control in how often they show up. Our brains are consistently producing thoughts, regardless of our attention or desire for them. So, while you might be able to silence your inner dialogue temporarily, the ability to not focus on anything in particular still remains an impossible task.

We can even test this right now.

Try to stop your thinking before you flip to the next page. Take a second to attempt to silence your thoughts now. Once you feel confident in your attempt, flip the page.

Notice how even if you wanted to, thoughts just show up. Now I want you to try and observe the type of thoughts that come to mind. So take a second to find a photo of someone you don't know on an advertisement. Make eye contact with the photo for one minute. Then come back and flip to the next page.

What did you notice with both exercises? Were you able to stop your thoughts? When looking at their face, you probably noticed thoughts show up as judgments as to who they might be or assumptions as to what they are like in person. How much did you or did you not like their face?

Just as we addressed in the last section, our brains automatically create thoughts to attach meaning to the content in our life. So, you couldn't stop your thoughts in the first exercise as they automatically placed meaning to the picture. These thoughts are out of our control. This brings up the first fundamental point in this book: that your inability to stop your thoughts is not a defect of your focus or ability, but rather a normal demonstration of how our biology influences our minds. How it is not us choosing to think thoughts, but rather us having to think. Simply put,

We do not have thoughts, thoughts have us.

They have you, me, and everyone else in the fact that we do not get a say in when they show up. We have to experience them regardless of if we close our eyes, try to change them, silence them, confirm them, or just watch them. Just as when you looked at the person's face in the exercise and started to think about who they might be like or how bizarre the exercise was. Thoughts compulsively appear as assessments and judgments to help us make sense of what we see, hear, and experience. Whether we dedicate a lifetime to silencing them through meditation, or a lifetime of trying to ignore the bad ones. These thoughts will always show up because we are biologically wired to need an understanding of the world around us. Like trying to hold your breath only to gasp back into breathing, this is part of what makes us human. Just as you would not try to remove your sex drive or the impulse to retract your hand away from something hot, our efforts are better spent understanding thoughts rather than controlling them.

In order to understand our thoughts, we have to first realize that our thoughts are not us; that in order to even experience them in our head, there has to be an experiencer for these thoughts to appear for. But this only becomes clear when you detach the thoughts that show up from the "*you*" I refer to, and the "*I*" you think in.

That means:

- The ideas you get about how to change your circumstances
- The logic and reasoning you use to justify behaviors
- The questions that show up about the intention and meaning of things
- The apparently accurate judgments and observations we have
- The opinions and assessments we conclude about situations
- The internal dialogue of stories about the drama of your life
- The concepts we identify with and take pride in

These, just to name a few variations of thought, are not you. They are automatically assigned thoughts that show up as a result of an internal need to make sense of the world that we will explore in depth later. What's important to understand is that these thoughts are coming from somewhere. That somewhere is what we will call a context.

| THE CONTEXT OF LIFE |

Context is everything. You often hear someone refer to something being taken out of context or needing context to explain something. This is because there is a series of agreed upon themes or topics that present the content in an intended form.

But in our case, there is not an agreed-upon context, rather a universally common one running in the background of our minds. It is a setting in which the contents of our lives are addressed within. This context forms a bias for the type of thoughts we get.

Context is directly responsible for the type of ways our thoughts appear. It could cause you to justify an experience that acts as a rationale for why you behave or feel a certain way, beliefs about ourselves or certain people we hold on to, and the meanings we place and refer to from past experiences. It is the source of what drives the rules and reasoning we buy into, who we are, and the ideas of how to get what we want. This context also hides under the guise of "smart thinking" and "best practices" for ways to avoid failure or pain, producing thoughts that appear as practicality or logic.

While context can serve us, the large majority of people are stuck with it silently running their lives without awareness of it. They have been experiencing it their whole lives, creating rules and ways of being that they have just gotten used to but never questioned the origins of. Because this context has been running for so long, an identity starts to shape around it.

This identity acts as a predictable way of hiding from the snake of our life. Be it the provider, caretaker, achiever, victim, oppressed, helper, comedian, teacher, lover, fighter, leader, supporter, or whatever else you identify with. This identity has become so second nature that you have likely forgotten a version of yourself that was free from this context.

Finish this sentence multiple times:

"I am a ______________________________"
"I am a ______________________________"
"I am a ______________________________"
"I am a ______________________________"

Whether you take pride in this list or not, what is important is not the roles we take but how those roles take us. This is because your answers are likely the identities you have grown comfortable with as a way to justify your decisions, actions, and life. The issue with this is that while an identity is validating, it also needs to be upheld in order to continue justifying our existence. That need produces never-ending obligations that control our life. Think of the achiever who takes pride in their accomplishments and receives validation for being that way, only to have that identity be expected from them because it is how people have come to accept them. They then make achievement a never-ending obligation to uphold if they want to be accepted.

Additionally, these identities contain a collection of thoughts and meanings that present the rules we have to live by. Such as the things you believe you need in order to be happy. The rule that once you get into that perfect relationship, then you will give it your all and be happy. Or once you get the dream job, car, house, or family, for your particular identity's needs, then you can be happy. These are nothing more than limitations on the emotions we are allowed to experience.

So, while this might just seem like a very normal way to exist in life, when we allow ourselves to look at our life from a fresh perspective, free from identities, obligations, rules, and the limiting roles we play, we can see what we are missing. When this happens, we become open to new chapters, outcomes, meanings, and possibilities. Experiencing a fresh start in our lives. It is from this place that we can find purpose, motivation, and happiness in life.

This is why we need to understand the effect context has on our life. Not just for the freedom we get from our limiting identities, but for the sake of truly maximizing how we spend time in this life.

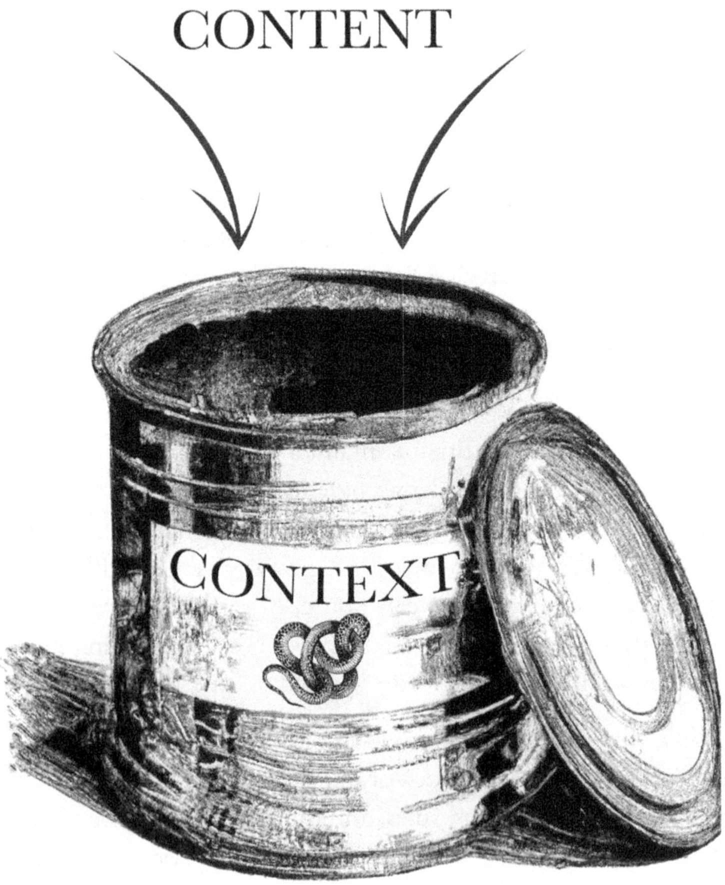
CONTENT
CONTEXT

| THE PAINT BUCKET OF CONTEXT |

The best way to see context is like an open paint bucket. Anything that goes into the bucket gets coated in paint. Let's say our paint bucket is full of red paint. Well, it doesn't matter if you throw a ring, coin, or key in there. All of those items will be painted red.

Similarly, our thoughts are the meaning that paints over the content of our life with the color from that bucket. So, it does not matter if you throw in a new relationship, different financial situation, or material possession; those circumstances are getting painted with meaning. This is how context controls our experience. It automatically contains a color in which our thoughts have to experience content with. So, if that paint bucket contains a color of dissatisfaction, the thoughts that show up to paint the content are all dissatisfied meanings.

While it is difficult to imagine how we could be dissatisfied with new circumstances like finally getting a dream job, this contextual paint will cover every bit of content you experience. Eventually, coating that dream job with unexpected annoyances, disrespectful coworkers, unfair demands, or limited opportunities. This is why changing the content of your life rarely improves the quality of your experience permanently. Also, this is why just changing thoughts rarely solves problems because it's like hoping not to get paint on something when it falls into the bucket. The only solution then is to change the paint bucket we use, which is the context.

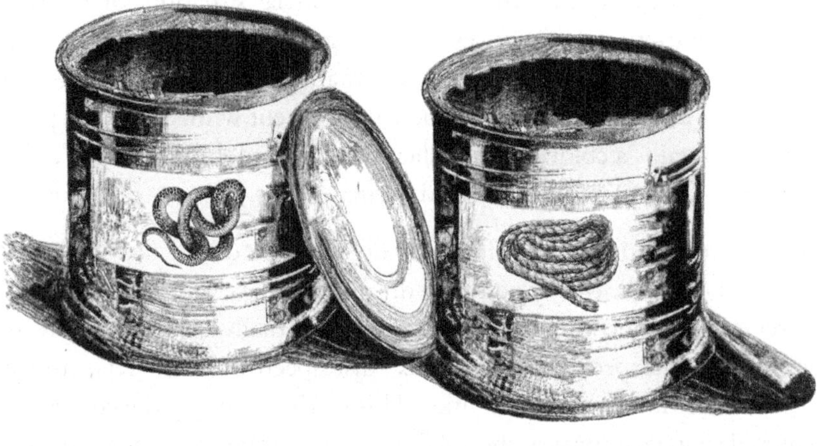

| THE TRUTH ABOUT THE SNAKE |

In my opinion, there are really only two types of paint buckets or contexts.

One is our default context and the other is a proactive context which will be explored in part three of this book. Our default context is based on our biology's survival wiring - which is why we default to it. By understanding it, we can shine a light on how it runs our daily life. This context has the colors of scarcity, shame, danger, fear, and dissatisfaction. If you have not guessed by now,

The snake in your life is your survival-based context.

It is the thing we are afraid to face and spend our time trying to avoid. It is the reason we live our lives as we do. At our core, we are wired to survive by any means necessary. Survival to us is any way in which our needs are met both biologically and psychologically.

So, it could start from a fear of abandonment that develops into an insecurity around not being worthy of love. This leads to having to uphold an inauthentic identity in relationships. Using this example, people may display behaviors such as compulsive lying to overcompensate value, all in an effort to avoid facing abandonment. This unfolding series of petty or embarrassing traits exists in all of us in one form or another and will be explored in greater depth in part two.

However, for now, all we need to do is understand that our default context is fueled by insecurity and fear that is a by-product of our need to survive. It is the snake we believe will be the death of us if we face. But through understanding the mechanisms that run our lives, we shine a light on our snakes and realize they are nothing more than ropes. So, let's start by understanding what exactly drives this default survival context.

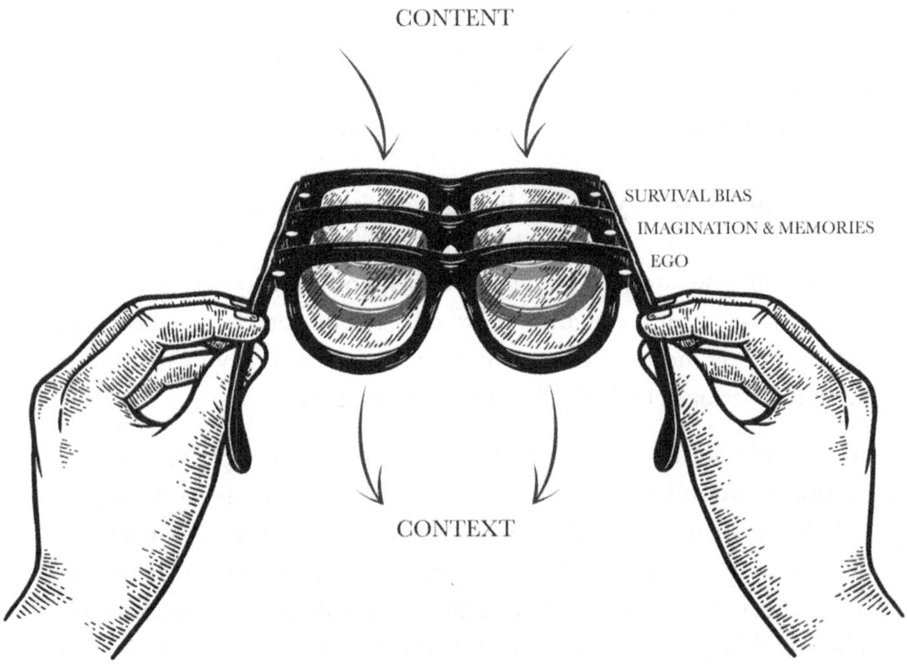
CONTENT
SURVIVAL BIAS
IMAGINATION & MEMORIES
EGO
CONTEXT

CHAPTER THREE
HUMAN BEINGS

| SURVIVAL BIAS |

We have evolved from very scarce and limited environments where the basic goal of survival was our only focus in life. This is no longer the case as we have developed out of the food chain and into more civilized environments. Regardless, the biological wiring that helped us adapt from that environment still operates within us. One of the ways this survival context messes with us is by constantly taking measurement and audit of what is possible or available within our current circumstance. So you measure your current financial situation against the job you already have, judge the availability of potential mates against everyone you already know, and imagine the range of enjoyment in life against your current habits. When this happens, we lock ourselves in a prison of limitation and scarcity, but we do this because our survival context can only measure what it can see, not the unlimited potential of possibility.

This also means:

You can only ever see what you will lose from any outcome, not what is possible to gain.

This is just one of the ways this survival context inhibits your perception and has you making scarcity-based decisions. As a result of this, you might find yourself over-concerned with what you can lose, miss out on, or not get from a situation. Which can have us holding on to unfulfilling jobs, incapable partners, and unsupportive friends, all because we cannot see the possibilities available to us when we make room for better outcomes.

It is this survival context that produces thoughts of limitation and scarcity in our lives when we are not aware of it. This is hardwired in us to do and is psychologically addictive to defend. Therefore, you, me, and everyone else naturally do this unless we are proactive against it.

You have probably heard the expression, "we are creatures of habit", but what that really means is that we are not wired for change. This is another part of our survival context because when life changes, we cannot predict it. The biological animal in us needs to predict life in order to feel safe. This survival wiring can be described as four traits:

1) Avoidance of pain

2) Seeking of pleasure

3) Maximizing these occurrences

4) Minimizing the effort to get them

From this, a series of mental mechanisms show up to help accomplish these goals.

- **The Ego:** This navigates, rationalizes, and defends these mechanisms, and the contents of our mind.

- **Our Memory:** This records and recalls all of the past experiences we have.

- **Our Imagination:** This uses the content of our memory to create future predictions

- **A Meaning Mechanism:** This makes associations and connections between the physical and mental.

While many books could be and have been written on any one of these mechanisms, the objective is to get a large viewpoint and basic understanding of how all of them create the thoughts that show up in our lives.

| EGO |

The simplest way to view the ego in relation to our mind is this: our ego uses our meaning mechanism, memory, and imagination to create and maintain the beliefs, identities, and lifestyles that aid in our need for survival and sex.

However, there are typically two competing streams of thought in the field of human potential and self-actualization on the ego:

> **1)** Ego is the problem of your existence; it is the reason you are superficial, never satisfied, and always want more. It is why you would rather be right than happy. It's the reason you get defensive with people and ideas that contradict you. It refuses valuable opportunities over maintaining pride and compulsively justifies unethical behavior like lying, stealing, and selfishness to secure its own survival. In essence, it is the poison of your life.
>
> **2)** Ego is the power of your experience. The fact that you are never satisfied with what you have, where you are, and your results in life is your human desire to keep advancing. It is what energizes you to keep experiencing more life, propelling you and our species forward. It is an eternal craving for more that keeps life interesting and enjoyable. This insatiable desire that keeps giving you opportunities to grow brings the happiness you want in life.

The thing about these conclusions is they both appear valid and logical. This is because the mechanisms that are able to make these judgments are designed to do just that: place meaning to things, making them good or bad. Regardless, we have to take a detached look at the ego as neither a good nor bad thing; it is simply content that we are painting. It is best to understand our ego as a tool of the mind, a very powerful system designed to heal, protect, and motivate us. It is a by-product of our psychology, so instead of trying to remove or increase it, we just need to understand it for what it is: the mechanism that allows for movement in our minds.

Part of the way it does this is by creating thoughts that defend our beliefs, ways of being, rules, and justifies our fears and insecurities. It allows us to do this so we can operate with confidence in our predictions on how to keep safe. It looks at the experiences we have survived and rationalizes them as the superior way of being. On one side, it closes us off to life, but on the other, it defends us against potentially dangerous outcomes. Its proclivity is to maintain itself and survive by defending the thoughts, actions, and feelings we have.

This shows up in almost all of our interactions with other people. Take for example having an argument with your significant other. Almost all arguments involve the interaction of two competing egos. You will recognize this if you have ever wanted to win an argument more than you wanted to accept differences or find common ground. This desire creates a need to get the other person to agree with your perspective or to see your rationale and clear-headed logic. Just as you feel this pressure to be right, they do too, which starts a back-and-forth discussion that soon evolves into a tense conflict as the exchange of ideas becomes more heated. This then escalates the conversation into other heated topics that are unrelated to the initial conversation. As this happens, we tend to become even more defensive and angry. This causes us to use hurtful language and take hostile jabs at the person's identity as a way to discredit their logic. At this point, we have likely forgotten what we were arguing about but just know we have to win. These experiences commonly end with both partners feeling defensive, angry, and unheard. Yet, regardless of how unproductive these conversations are, our egos are continually ready to engage in an endless amount of them.

These are the moments when we find our ego causing us to repeat disempowering thought patterns, toxic habits, and stubbornness in the face of potentially productive outcomes. Alternatively, our ego motivates us with grandiose images of success and visions of our importance and value to the world, enabling us to surpass our fears and improve our lives. It also rejects the criticism and unproductive opinions of other people in favor of believing its own narratives. This allows us to be critical of ideas and protect ourselves from being helplessly gullible and susceptible to the will of other people's survival needs over our own.

All of these examples happen because our ego is designed to be right. As a result of being right, we receive dopamine, which gives us a sense of security about our worldview and our lives. This is very addicting to our nervous system and biology because it is at the root of our survival wiring. In order to accomplish all of this, our ego takes advantage of our mind and other mechanisms that we will explore next.

| IMAGINATION & MEMORY |

Our mind is composed of two very powerful tools that together are uniquely human:

1) The ability to vividly remember the past

2) The ability to vividly imagine the future

These abilities, if used correctly, allow us to use our past to make better decisions and allow our imagination to craft motivating futures for us to strive towards. But if misused or unused, it can cause us fear, anxiety, depression, and nearly all the dissatisfaction we experience. In fact, if we do not successfully manage these abilities, they tend to manage us.

When this happens, they tend to first show up as paranoid or fearful thoughts that paint painful or dangerous outcomes that could occur. For example, we might imagine the embarrassment we would feel if we got rejected or failed. We then interpret these thoughts as accurate predictions or assessments of the situation at hand. This continues over and over until these thoughts craft the rules and guidelines we use to avoid the snake in our analogy, which ultimately makes up our lives.

These predictions and assessments seem valid because our imagination pulls from our memory which contains the ability to vividly experience pain from our past. When this happens it is like painting over all-new content with a painful experience, causing us to relive painful experiences despite having new relationships, jobs, or circumstances. Additionally, we are imagining an endless stream of possible ways for different painful experiences to occur should the circumstances change.

You can really observe your imagination and memory in action with our ability to create excuses for why you cannot do something that you have been putting off. Take any tedious chores you remember disliking, such as:

- Doing your taxes
- Going to the gym
- Cleaning your home or car
- Preparing your meals
- Doing your laundry
- Starting a new work project

You will notice that you are able to create endless amounts of excuses as to why "now is not a good time" or how something else is more critical when really it is not. This is because our mind has an imagination that is capable of endless reasons, logic, excuses, and apparent truths to keep us feeling the way we feel. Our minds are not in the business of being changed; they are in the business of staying the same and surviving. As a result, anything that could potentially advance us or change us is often met with resistance. Remember these mechanisms are just a product of a biological need to feel safe. So when we are presented with anything that could change us, our mind fills in the gaps with thoughts that our imagination and memory has cooked up. The problem comes when we begin to accept those thoughts as reasonable, logical, and apparently true assessments that know better.

| MEANING |

All of these mechanisms work together to create the thoughts that communicate the meaning we place to content. It is our mind's job to fill in that gap between the external stimulus and its relation to us. Since we are fundamentally wired to not accept randomness, a meaning must be filled. If something happens, we want to know why as it lets us know how to avoid pain and gain pleasure. Just think of how drawn you are to the sight of a car accident on the side of the road. It is the negative associations we have to the lights of an ambulance, firetruck, or police car that make us want to understand the meaning behind what caused it. It is very difficult for us to just experience something as it is without attaching meaning. As a result, we automatically fill the gap with an interpretation aligned with our survival-based context. This is what makes us think the person must have been driving drunk, on their phone, or not paying attention. We need to try and make sense of things to help us avoid similar experiences.

While it is a tough pill to swallow, it is through this process that we have unintentionally experienced our life. Meaning, importance, and value we attribute to things are usually just a collection of biased opinions. All of which come from default contexts our psychologies use for biological survival. That is all. Whether we accept this or not, the evidence of this is clear once we are honest with ourselves about why we do what we do, which is what part two is all about. So, this now brings us to the last section of part one which begins to unpack exactly how we stop our survival-based context from being our default.

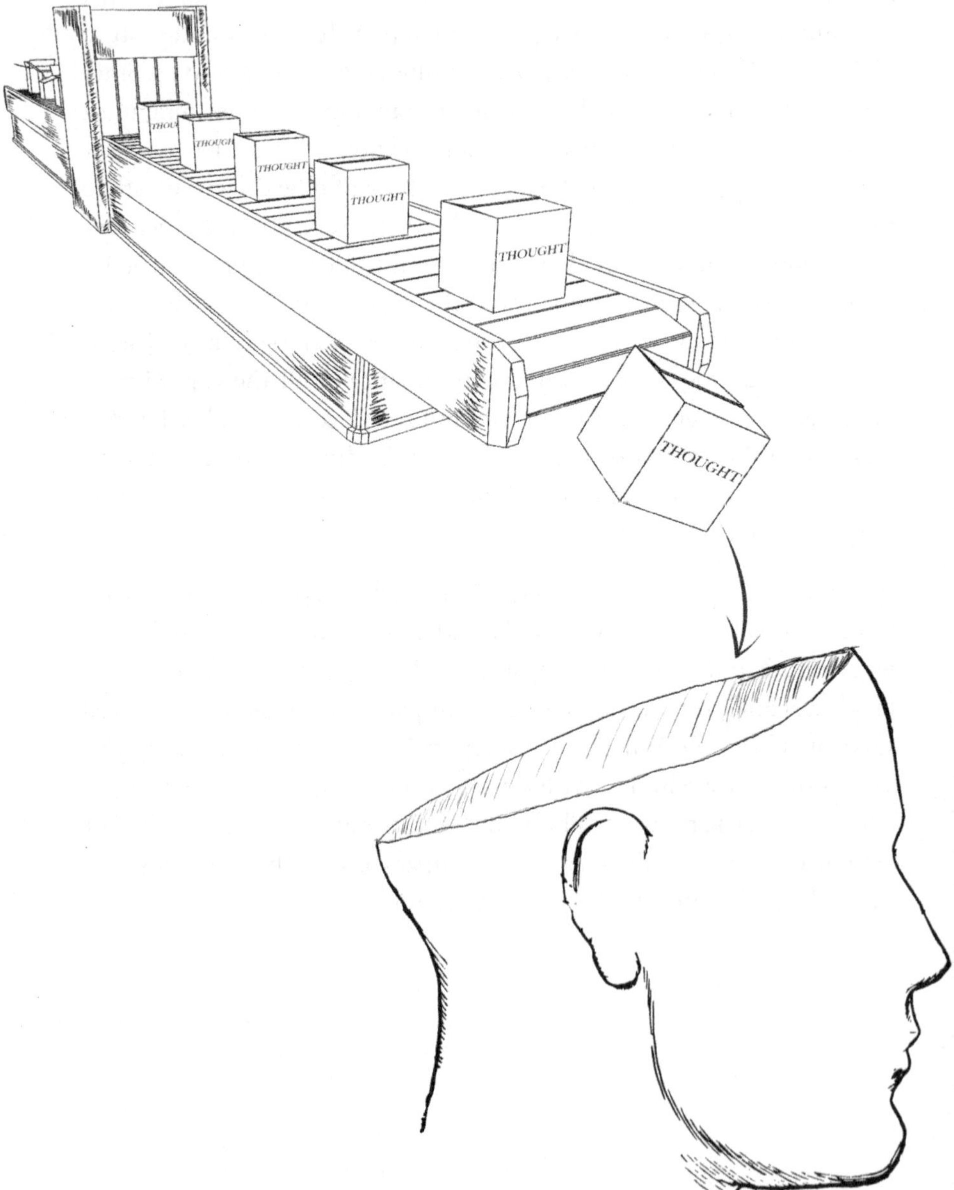
THOUGHT
THOUGHT
THOUGHT
THOUGHT
THOUGHT
THOUGHT

CHAPTER FOUR
AWARE

| MEETING YOURSELF |

When asked the question of who you are, you'll often refer to your body, name, job, group identity, or some variation of that, such as:

- "I am a gender"
- "I am name"
- "I am a profession"
- "I am a belief"
- "I am a role"
- "I am a behavior"
- "I am a personality trait"

However, when we narrow down the question to who the "I" is that you are referring to in your answer, things get a little trickier. Take for example your own answers:

Who are you?

I am ______________________________

I am ______________________________

I am ______________________________

I am ______________________________

I am ______________________________

Now with your answers, try to point to who the "I" is in those statements, without relying on the adjectives used after "I am"

Can you identify and point to the "you" this book refers to?

Who is the "I" in that statement?

The quickest answer that most people will point to is their thoughts or inner dialogue. But as we have previously explored, those thoughts and inner dialogues are just reactions to our biology, ego, and social conditioning. None of which are uniquely us that we can point to as a source of who we are. This is because,

You are not your thoughts, you are only the observer who watches the thoughts come in.

So, this returns us back to the question of who exactly is the "I" that we refer to and live our lives as.

The "I" that experiences the thoughts and our life as it's being lived is an observer.

Simply put, you are an observer of your life. It is not necessarily a thing we can point to as who we are, but instead it is a quality in us that is able to observe and be aware. So it's not the beliefs, thoughts, or identity we think in, rather it is the sensation of distance between the vivid experience of having a thought versus thought as an object.

It is important to not see the observer as an entity or subject separate from us - it is us. Our survival context often has us thinking that it is another thought we can point to. If this happens, remember that this is more of an internal sensation of awareness than a concept or thought. It can help to go back to the question of:

Who is the "I", in "I am"?

Without trying to come up with an answer you can point to, just experience the question as a sensation. Experience the question as a space you can stand in and feel. That is you, without context.

If this is still confusing, that is quite ok. Coming face to face with yourself as an observer is a skill set. Like being a detached scientist who studies something, only you study your own thoughts. While this might seem nuanced and complicated, do not worry if you are still not getting it. Part two of this book has been designed to help you come face to face with "I", so that you can experience being an observer in relation to all the different areas of your life. For now, this was important to bring up so that we can understand what allows us to stop living from our survival context, which is to observe and become aware.

| DISTINCTIONS & AWARENESS |

The actual process of observing or creating self-awareness starts by knowing what to look for against something else. This is known as a distinction. A distinction is the ability to differentiate between two things.

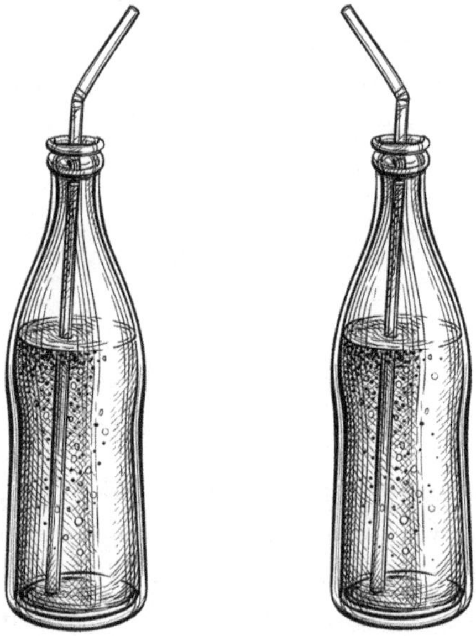

Take for example Pepsi versus Coca-Cola. To those who drink cola, these are completely different, while to someone who does not drink soda, they are both just cola. Well, why is this important?

It is in our distinctions that we gain awareness.

If someone changes their drink order if the restaurant does not serve their preference of cola, their distinction between the two colas has helped them pick out a more preferable experience. This can also happen with our context and the thoughts, emotions, and behaviors that come from them. Once we gain awareness of the different ingredients that make up the recipe of a context, we can choose to select a new context that serves us. Until then, they are chosen for us, like a person without soda distinctions ordering a cola. This is what observation and awareness are all about. The more awareness you have, the more choice you have.

Life is really about choice. The more you have, the better your experience in life will be.

So the goal of life is to fully control what we do have a choice in. As referred to earlier, human beings are creatures of habit. This means our default setting is to do what is most normal to us, which is to maintain our survival context.

When we default to this, we live life in an automatic setting with automatic thoughts, creating automatic emotions which cause automatic behaviors and decisions, producing similar outcomes that fuel more automatic thinking. If our thoughts are just the by-products of how our environment and past experiences have taught us how to avoid pain and gain pleasure, then your purpose, meanings, feelings, relationships, and available opportunities are out of your control. This makes your life based entirely on your survival context and what you learned from your environment and past experiences.

This is why the majority of people live similar lives to their parents and peers. The only thing that allows an individual to stop acting, feeling, and thinking automatically is awareness. If you do not understand why you feel what you feel, why you have always had bad relationships, or why you have the outcomes you have in life, that is a sign that it is being automatically chosen for you. Thus, you do not have awareness of the distinctions that cause it. This means that anything you are not aware of, you do not have control or choice over.

Think of an infant who can't move their head. They have no control over what they see until they become aware of their muscles and motor skills. This means they have no choice in what they view or where they go, making their vision and location in the automatic setting. At one point in our childhood, we became aware of the thoughts in our heads.

When this happened, we no longer just randomly and unconsciously thought. Instead, we had control over what we wanted to focus on, and that awareness allowed us to choose what to focus on.

Then as we grew up into teenagers, we became aware that other people had thoughts that feel just as important to them as ours do to us. This allowed us to influence and connect with people as we became aware of their likely desires and values, thus giving us a choice in how we relate and react to other people.

In the same way, when you start to become aware of the different distinctions and patterns that control your emotions, you can start selecting and controlling the emotions and behaviors that were once automatic.

Most people do not have awareness of what is controlling their lives which is why they do not believe they can take control of their own lives.

The primary goal of this book is to help you gain awareness into the ontology of your life, which is to be aware of how you actually live your life, not how your thoughts make you think you are living it. This is how we shine a light on the snake that is our survival context.

| OBSERVATION |

So, in order to control this survival context, we have to start with an awareness of it. This is done by observing it, and observation requires two things.

1) First, the individual needs to take 100% responsibility for their life.

You cannot observe what is going on internally until you stop looking for external excuses. When you believe your life is the by-product of external factors like other people, environments, and circumstantial content, you inadvertently hand over your control to them. Even if it is influenced by external factors, awareness requires us to suspend the possibility that something else is causing our outcomes. We need to operate, even just temporarily, with the acceptance of every outcome in our life being our responsibility. Part two will help you do this in more detail.

2) The second thing that allows for observation is distinctions.

You need to know what to look for if you want to observe it. This is the easy part if you have read up to here because that is exactly what this book has explored so far. It is why the prior pages educated you on the different mechanisms that make up your mind and life. Just by reading about how your psychology and inner workings create your experience, you have already learned the distinctions of what to look for in others and yourself.

| WHAT HAPPENS NOW? |

Here is what you can expect so far. If you have been reading this and engaging with the ideas and genuinely trying to apply them to your own life, you probably noticed having a couple of "ah-ha" or "woah" moments. If so, thank you for taking 100% responsibility. It was your willingness to accept that this is something you are doing to yourself combined with the distinctions of how you go about doing it that made those "ah-ha" moments possible. When those moments hit, you most likely felt a profound feeling of insight as you became aware of how your survival context influenced your life. While likely nothing has changed about your life just yet, you did become aware of why you have the outcomes and experiences you have.

That sensation is just a glimpse of what it is like to shine a light on the snake in your life. In that brief glimpse, your awareness returned to you as the observer of your life, making you free from directly experiencing the outcome you reassessed. In that moment, you detached from the survival context and had an opportunity to choose a new context for that content. Again, it was only for a brief moment, but this is how it starts.

If you have not yet had one of these moments but are still reading, thank you for your continued interest. What happens for a lot of people that learn this is that it hits them while they are naturally going about their day. So, as you close these pages, put this book down, and carry on with your life, you will have a thought come into your mind that sparks your memory of reading about how this type of thought happens. It may be in the form of a judgment you make towards someone, like having someone cut in front of you while driving assuming they did it on purpose. Then, you consider the possibility that perhaps they are late for a job interview. As this happens, the realization hits you that you are placing meaning as a need to make sense of the world, not as an objective assessment of the situation.

Regardless of where you are at with the book so far, when you gain awareness of the survival context in your life, a gap is created between the automatically chosen context and the content without context. This is an opportunity to disengage from content that once caused pain, which is like viewing the content without the paint of context or using that opportunity to re-engage with a better context for enjoyment. This is like changing the paint bucket to produce a more pleasurable meaning - but more on these options later.

Just as we learned before, when a person learns how to avoid more pain or gain more pleasure, they will automatically choose that option every time. This is how you increase your awareness through observation, and with that, how you change your life.

| PREFACE FOR PART II |

Part one was about the nature of our existence and how it causes problems. In part two, we do not just take a distanced look at these issues, we rather get up close and face them head-on.

See, if we are genuinely interested in turning a light on to expose the snake of our own life, we need to be honest about the degree to which it has affected us in all areas of life - even the ones we are proud of. It is one thing to read about an imagined snake that influences our life, but it is another thing to actively hunt for the light switch by being honest about your inauthenticity and misperceiving nature.

It is important to understand that while the intensity and tone of this book will change to a harsher one in part two, it is for the sole purpose of helping you face what almost no one is willing to face. It is not my intention to belittle your challenges or discredit your life in any way that places me above you. Rather, it is with great respect and dignity that I have the opportunity to invite you to turn a light on alongside me continually turning on my own. So with that said, it is time for us to find some rope.

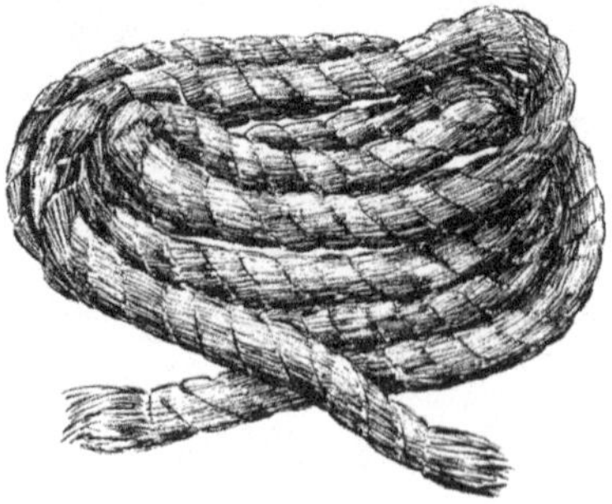

PART II

LIFE & BEING

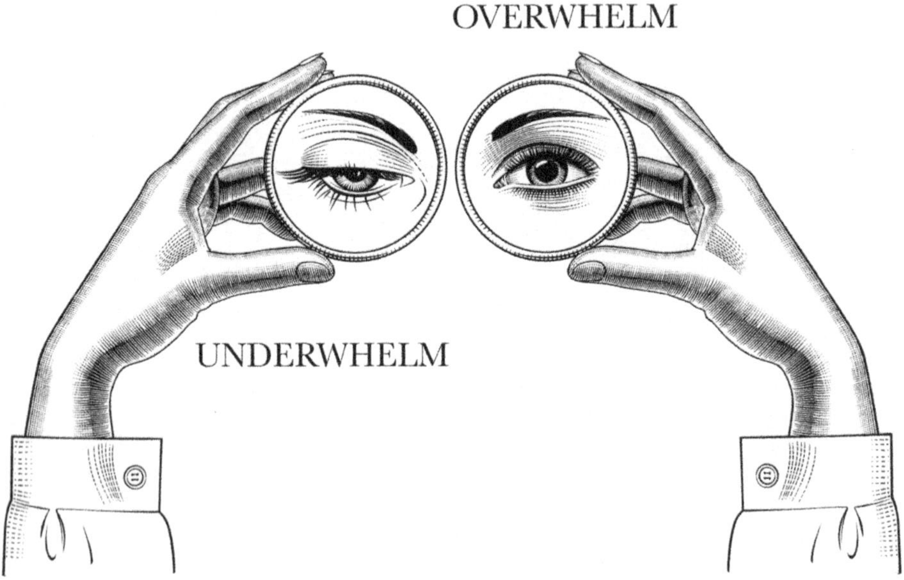
OVERWHELM
UNDERWHELM

CHAPTER FIVE

HOW LIFE UNFOLDS

| UNDERWHELM & OVERWHELM |

After years of study, late nights, and sacrificed social events, a young woman finally lands the job of her dreams at the ideal law firm she wanted after graduating from university. Everyone around her congratulates and praises the ambition and focus that led her there. Her parents are full of pride as they tell their co-workers, friends, and extended family of her accomplishment. By most people's estimations, she should be glowing with excitement. Yet to her surprise, she feels a certain emptiness with this experience, almost as though the conversations and celebrations seem to glaze past her in a dream-like fashion. She interprets this underwhelming reaction as not feeling it's real, but more than this, it is that the emotion she thought she would have is not registering.

This sensation of underwhelm seems to continue until a feeling of overwhelm arises and carries her into the new job, new office, and day-to-day habits she now has to adjust to - all of which she justifies to herself as just getting the hang of things. Once she no longer feels overwhelmed with all the changes in her life, she is met once again with a feeling of underwhelm. She gets a sensation of finality that starts to sink in as she comes face to face with the imagery that pushed her years before. But like graduation, it is more of a feeling of trying to catch up with an emotion that is not there, like trying to walk up close to a fog that seems to clear itself as one approaches.

Time moves on and she is now caught up with trying to maintain her praise as a lawyer and the demands that come with her career. This sensation of trying to catch up or get ahead then starts to become a consistent theme in her life, either financially with the new lifestyle this job afforded or with the workload of her now long-term career. Just as one thing seems to be handled, she notices another issue arising, be it a little weight gain, lack of a love life, or even just an annoyance at work. There never seems to be a moment of pause to stop and take in her life as it unfolds.

As the years go on, her life appears to be a mix between feeling overwhelmed and underwhelmed, but never just content. Yet she continually believes that there will be a time in the future when things can be this way, where things just work and exist without a rush, allowing her to just be. One belief after another shows up as something to look forward to next, like when she gets to travel, get married, get that house on the lake, get promoted to partner, get to be a mother, and so on. But still, as life progresses and these supposedly celebratory or desired moments occur, she is again met with similar feelings of underwhelm and overwhelm and she is always consumed with the responsibilities and challenges that stand in front of her. When asked about her experiences, she describes them as how she imagined them, not taking into account that her actual experience of them felt distracted with that feeling of being in her head and trying to process what she was going through.

| DREAMS, GOALS & MILESTONES |

This story is not unique. It is happening to all of us in all elements of our lives, from big things like our work and relationships to small things like waiting for a package in the mail. This is how our lives tend to unfold, as a series of moments containing overwhelm and underwhelm. Never truly getting an opportunity to reach a place in life where we feel content and in total control. In one moment, we were consumed with the stress of a situation like finances or living arrangements. Next, we are bored and feel empty at the apparent mundaneness and repetition of our lives, craving some distant achievement. One side of us craves a future in which we can just decompress and relax for a moment, yet another side yearns for a better future that has more luxurious circumstances.

Even though almost all moments contain either of these sensations, we tend to defend and advertise our lives by highlighting the accomplishments that we have achieved to justify the suffering that was required to obtain them. Or perhaps we are trying to convince ourselves to feel the emotions those milestones were supposed to provide us.

Be it university, marriage, having kids, working in a particular industry, or traveling to name a few. The actual experience of these things, moment to moment, is very different than the idea of what they are like in retrospect. Despite this, we promote them as undeniably enjoyable experiences that everyone should experience. Now, this is not to suggest that these things cannot be pleasurable. Instead, there is a difference between the pleasure we get from the thought of how those experiences unfold versus actually experiencing them. One is a mental movie which highlights scenes of the experience unfolding. The other is the attention we maintain from moment to moment, like you have right now, as your inner dialogue reads each word in this sentence out loud to you in your mind - that internal attention that is just focused on the present and its sensations.

We rarely hear about this difference because it is automatically hidden from us, as we live under the rules and rationalizations our mind makes. While there are many rationalizations, the most common ones you might be thinking of as you read this is:

"I could see how other people do this but I am different"

or

"This makes sense but my situation is unique"

The only reason you might believe this does not affect you is because you are actually unaware of how in-depth and involved these mechanisms are in our lives. That thought alone is nothing more than the defense mechanism of our ego trying to prevent us from changing. It uses rationalized inner dialogue as an attempt to discredit what you are reading as irrelevant to you. But as we explored in part one, those thoughts are not us. Our nervous system has been designed to do this regardless of our wishes. This means, you, me, and everyone else that is human is affected by this, regardless of our personal or cultural differences. So, I encourage you to at least entertain the possibility that these topics are very much about you, regardless of the automatically defensive thoughts that show up against them.

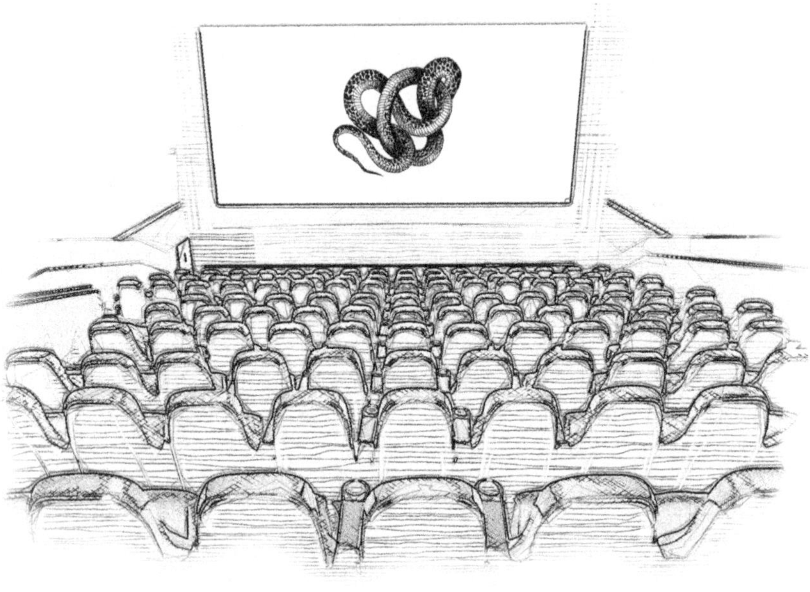

| THE MOVIE OF LIFE |

Many of us think that our life is similar to a movie in that there are main characters, side characters, and enemies all interacting and navigating through the ups and downs of a plot. In which, hardships and challenges ultimately lead to success or failure, like the young woman who got her ideal job after years of hard work at university. But the fact of the matter is that the thoughts that create the movie plot of our lives do so regardless of the events that occur within our movie.

Take any painful or difficult event from your past right now.

How do you think that led you to where you are right now?

How does that relate to the bigger picture of your life?

Your answers are your mind creating the movie you believe your life is about. But the issue with this movie is that you never actually see the conclusion of it. Instead, you are only ever living right before the good part happens. Perhaps you studied hard at university yet still failed and then dropped out. Your mind tells the story of the dropout who will make a comeback later with business. Or how it was not until you dropped out that you realized what you were actually passionate about. Or how dropping out and getting a job led you to meet the love of your life. Or any variation of a story in which the experience of dropping out is justified in the bigger picture of a better outcome that will unfold in the future. Either way, this movie keeps changing as it is being watched.

The reality is that dropping out of university is neither good nor bad. There is no hidden meaning or story behind it and it is not a plot point in the epic movie of your life.

Your past is just something that happened in which you observed and experienced.

While you might feel defensive about this idea, it is only because we use these movies to justify the previous suffering and pain we have gone through. But as explained in part one, this defensiveness is just our automatic function of placing meaning to things that makes us believe it is part of a greater story. Then our ego defends that story as a way to help us rationalize that suffering. When this happens, we can understand that pain in relation to how we think things will work out. Thus, we can use that interpretation as a basis for future decisions in order to try to avoid similar pain in the future. Needless to say, we are very invested and attached to these movies because they feel like the bases for the point of our lives up to now.

So, we really want to examine this attachment to our thoughts and the movies they create. Not so we can live without them like cold and detached robots without emotions. Instead, we can actually experience the very thing we believe our storytelling and justifying will lead us to, a state of contentment, free from underwhelm or overwhelm.

Think about something you hope will pan out for you in the future, something that you have been going through or working towards.

As you imagine it, notice how you place your current situation and experience in relation to it. You judge your current situation as painful or annoying in some way and that future situation as pleasurable and free. What we are talking about is how much of our life is spent in a state of longing for the future while judging our current experience as one to get out of, and how your current circumstance only makes sense in the movie that contains the future situation.

But really think about this. If your life was actually a movie, you would not be able to know what type of movie you were living in. So while we tend to picture ourselves in a tragedy or hero story, neither could be known without a complete collection of all of our experiences packaged within a context of a happy or sad movie. This is because, in order for something to be a story, the events must already be laid out so we could define what type of story it was. Is it a romance, a comedy, or a thriller? That would all depend on the events that occurred. Did the hero achieve the goal or fail? Did they get romance or lose it?

In order for you to know what movie you are living in, you would have to know exactly how it all panned out. This is only truly possible once the movie ends, which in our case is death. So, there is no living version of you that is even capable of knowing what movie you are in. This means that the movie you think you are living in is nothing more than your mind using its mental mechanisms like memory, imagination, and the ego to give you the experience that you are playing out a meaningful story.

The harsh conclusion of this is that our lives are intrinsically meaningless. There is not an unfolding agenda or hidden story behind things. It is not that your past suffering means any more than your current experience. Things just are. They are not heading in any meaningful direction with some story that makes it all worth it. The reality of the matter is that:

Your life is not going to work out because it already has worked out. In that, you are living how it panned out *right now*.

You are currently living the full movie right now as you read these words because there was not a movie to begin with. Just the thoughts and internal story of one that shows up for us to observe. That movie might be the importance of your career, how serious or casual you believe your relationship is, the thoughts you tell yourself about how much people like or dislike you, or the perception of how relevant you are to a community or industry. Regardless, it is a story and collection of meanings that all of us, in one way or another, choose our lives around in an effort to either change or maintain our situation.

This is how we actually spend the majority of our time. Stuck in the meaningless mental movies we try to influence or maintain. Causing us to just "think" our life instead of actually living our life.

This looks a lot like us just overthinking about our job, relationships, and purpose in life, having thoughts about what we need to do or change, or what is right or wrong about any given situation. We think if we do not do this or that then people will think negatively of us. If we can just get that thing, we can then finally achieve or be a certain way. There are endless thoughts and variations of movies, but there is really one major theme that they all have in common:

Happiness comes.

It is this single belief that keeps us addicted to our movies and stuck in our own heads. It is a hope that one day we will be truly happy if X, Y, and Z happen. The truth is that happiness never comes. It is not a distant experience that you reach and forever exist in because just as you are experiencing the world right now with all of your mental movies, that is exactly how you will experience it later, with a similar movie that keeps happiness in the distance.

Your belief that you can in some way influence this by changing your circumstance is nothing more than you hiding from this snake. It is a lie. So much so that you think those brief moments of achievement or success are you experiencing happiness. When in actuality, they are just temporary moments in which you think you have avoided the snake, never taking the time to turn the light on and experience life without the compulsive need to get to the future. Until you realize this, you are forever suffering from imaginary snakes and movies that never actually pan out in your favor. The suffering and pain you experienced in your past will continue to cause you more suffering until you can accept that it is just our mind placing meaning and nothing more. Accept that life just happens without meaning until our mind paints it with a context that depicts it as bad. This traps us in internal fantasies of how to justify and fit that suffering into a movie where we end up happy. Until you get this, you only *think* your life instead of actually living it.

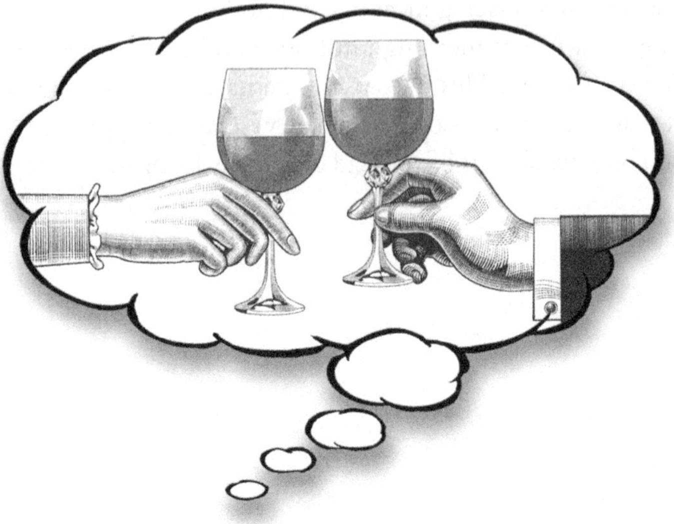

THINKING OUR LIFE
VS
EXPERIENCING OUR LIFE

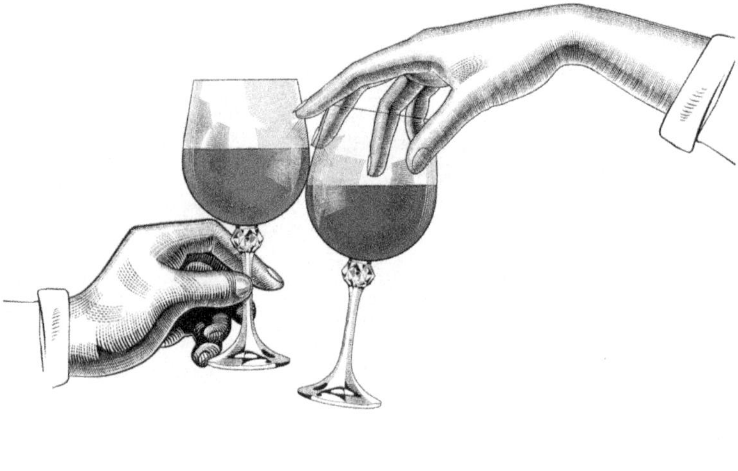

| MOVIES & EXPERIENCE |

The first light we need to turn on is how we actually spend our time. Not in the sense of how our time is scheduled with where we go and what we do. Instead, how we go through those actions internally with our minds. In part one, we recognized who we are as just observers and how we are not our thoughts, only the observation of them. The importance of this distinction is to recognize the difference and separation between the thoughts that create our mental movies and experience as it is without meaning.

Without this distinction, we confuse what is *experienced* in life versus what is *thought* about life. When this line in the sand is not drawn, our time in life is more often than not spent in our heads imagining movies. So to clarify this, we need to start with the difference between the statements:

"I love my partner" as a thought
versus
"Loving my partner" as an experience

While the statements are similar, they produce two very different outcomes. We know this because we can feel these statements show up differently in our life. One is a concept that we think and live through mentally. The other is an emotional state of being that is felt and commonly expressed physically. But, because we spend the majority of our time within these mental movies,

We *think* our life instead of *experiencing* our life.

While you may be able to recall moments when you were truly engaged in an experience in your life, it is safe to say that the majority of your life has been spent getting caught up in your thoughts as though the mental movies were real. But because these movies seem so real, we tend to base our decisions and lives around them. This causes us to just mentally live a movie called, "I love my partner," which feels like us trying to maintain, change, and work through issues, or fix or forgive something in the relationship. All of this is just an effort to get to some future where none of those issues exist. Where we can finally allow ourselves to love them as they are. But the movie never gets to that part, so we almost never actually experience "I love my partner." Instead, we only ever think about it.

This distinction becomes even clearer when we imagine how a random person would observe us interacting with our partner. What would they see if they had no background knowledge of the movies being lived by both people? They would not see the movie of trying to get to the bottom of that time when your partner hurt you, or how you both need to figure out where this relationship is heading. To that random person, the relationship is already figured out and it is just two people exchanging words. Spending their time together bickering and arguing mental movie outcomes. That is what it is, despite our belief that it is more. Being over-concerned with the completion of a movie that never actually comes true is how most people actually spend their time.

This is not a criticism of your particular relationship. Instead, it is an observation on the nature of how a large majority of people actually spend their time relating to one another. It is not just relationships in which these movies play out; it is in every single thing we believe is important in life. See, most people *think* their lives as they make up movies on how they believe their time is being spent. However, in actuality, their life contains almost none of the emotions or experiences that the movie attempts to express. Take for example the differences between these thoughts:

- "I love what I do" versus experiencing love through doing
- "I am happy in my job" versus experiencing happiness within the job
- "I have problems" versus experiencing moments of challenge among times without

- "People like when I do that" versus experiencing people react in a way that I perceive as likable

This difference is the key to spending your time well on this earth. Without it, our biological tendency to place meaning and force thoughts into our minds takes over our time and life. It fills us with mental movies and stories of how our life is going. It has us buy into illusions about our own importance and the seriousness of our relationships when actually, importance and seriousness are nothing but movies we buy into to make us feel safe about the future.

This happens so automatically for us that it has become near to impossible for most people to identify their life as anything outside of a mental movie. That can make this realization and distinction very uncomfortable to accept, but nevertheless, it is the harsh reality of how we spend our time.

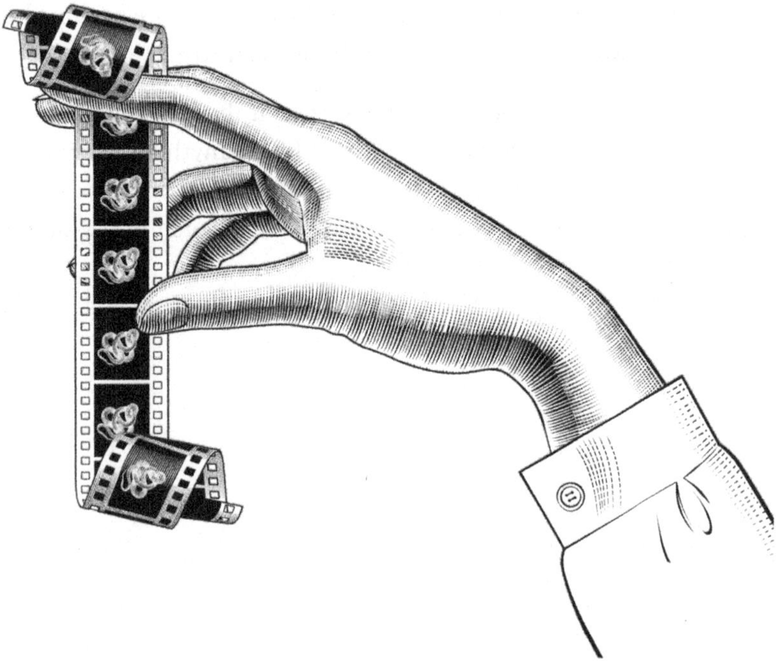

| STEPPING INTO THE PROJECTOR ROOM |

The reason we want to make this distinction is not because we want to live without mental movies, this is not possible as we described in part one. Rather, this distinction allows us to spend more time actually *experiencing* the emotions we desire, instead of just *thinking* that our time is being spent in that way. By doing so, we can make the reality of our lives more enjoyable, fulfilling, and purposeful.

One of the best ways to catch this in action is by noticing when our inner dialogue crafts the logic for our movies. See, when you are really enjoying yourself, totally consumed in the moment, fully experiencing the sensations of that situation, your thoughts, and inner dialogue are not there.

It is only when things become unpleasant, unfavorable, or uncomfortable that the 'I' that most people think in, tends to show up.

It is only when we are unhappy that we have thoughts about what is not okay, how it could be better, or what needs to change. Until that point, we just experience the flow of our work, or life as it is without meaning. Fully taking in the situation at hand. But because this is such a rare sensation for most people, they attempt to hold onto it by capturing it by thinking about it. Creating entire fantasies and mental movies around the moments they previously had. Holding these moments as sacred and valuable. As though the memory of those moments is in any way similar to actually experiencing them. Take for example a moment like:

- Loosing yourself in flirtation or passion with a partner
- A period of endless creativity where you lost track of time
- A feeling of deep curiosity or interest in which focus no longer seemed like a problem

For most people, these moments tend to be rare when compared to just the mental remembering of them, so they become our ideals and expectations. Yet, ironically by doing this, we inadvertently guarantee we will not get more of them. This is because, in order for those moments to have existed in the first place, they relied on our thoughts not being there to begin with.

| SO, WHAT'S THE POINT? |

If the goals of our movies never bring us happiness, what is the point of trying in life? Firstly, this is not a suggestion that a person just forfeits their life and denounces and neglects their responsibilities, disregards their health and desires, and adopts hedonism as their new way of being.

This realization is not a rationalization to no longer attempt to improve our lives.

Otherwise, what would be the point of even reading further. The point is to understand the place at which our actions and efforts come from. This will enable us to proactively observe our mind instead of just being the reaction of it. This ability to willfully observe our subjectivity distances us from the complaining and suffering that would have previously consumed us. It allows us to experience our efforts to improve our lives just as they are, meaningless behaviors that lead to different circumstances. From this proactive place, we can now enjoy the act itself, just as an experience, for the sake of doing it. Separate from the thoughts and fantasies that will still show up about how challenging or painful the process is. Simply put, we can enjoy improving for the sake of it without all the complaining. It is enjoying challenge and change for the pure reason that we have the opportunity to do so while on this earth.However, this is not to be confused with consciously suffering for a story or just reframing our pain in a positive light, like saying, "all these late nights of working will be worth it once I get promoted," or, "perhaps these sacrifices will help me gain the contrast needed to enjoy my life later." Both of these are like the example of our paint bucket from part one where someone who does that is really just painting things differently, yet still using the same paint color which is a context of dissatisfaction. It is through acceptance of this realization and returning to observation that we are able to either see things without the paint or change the paint bucket to a more deliberate one.

| SAVING OURSELVES |

Regardless of your awareness of these fantasies and movies playing out in your life, you will still notice you default to them. Part of this is because you have likely had a lifetime of living through your thoughts as though they were real. Therefore, it will take some time to just observe them. Another reason is that, as mentioned earlier, we are attached to these fantasies. We are invested in them coming true. Part of the way we try to increase the intensity and probability of them coming true is by saving ourselves.

This means we do not allow ourselves to just enjoy things for what they are. Instead, we reserve our good emotions and satisfied states for when we finally get the objective.

This looks like us actively maintaining a frustrated or dissatisfied state of being with the work we do and the people we are with. It is based on the premise that "I will only give my all when it matters. Until that point, I am saving my effort". We tell ourselves that we will work hard when the right opportunity shows up or when we get a raise or praise. Or, we talk about putting effort into a relationship only when the right person appears or when someone apologizes or acts the way we want. The issue with that is:

We do not get what we want in life; we get who we are.

Both the right opportunities and people come as a result of us being the type of person who already allows for those outcomes to appear.

So, if you are unmotivated when you work for someone else, you will most likely remain unmotivated once you work for yourself. If you cannot make yourself happy, you are not likely to keep someone who does make you happy.

We have to show up at the level that we want to receive in life.

This business of saving ourselves is critical to the overall happiness you receive in life. It is most commonly found in ourselves when we observe our rules for what makes us happy.

Look at what it takes for you to be happy. What are the series of outcomes and situations that have to occur in order for you to allow happiness to exist within you? Are you only happy when you have had a productive day? Does it require you to have gotten perfect sleep the night before, with zero frustrations in your day? While also having some unique surprises and variety that you weren't expecting?

So ask yourself now
"What does it take for me to have an amazing day?"

What I want you to notice is not the simplicity of the list but rather the size of it. Simplicity is often the result of our minds generalizing. So you might have said, "Any day I wake up early is an amazing day." Yet there are plenty of days when this simplistic answer did not cut it if we actually look back on how you spent that day moment by moment. So, it is not the simplicity of our answers but rather how few of them there are.

Now I want you to answer the question:
What kind of things could disrupt your day?

I want you to notice now how much larger that list is. Your mind probably had no difficulty thinking of the many different things you hate and find annoying. The result of this is that you have more ways to be unhappy than you do happy. This means the rules you set up for yourself on how to be happy are almost impossible to win.

The goal is not to tamper with our thoughts by trying to force out a larger list of things that make you happy. As we learned in part one, we are fighting against a mind and context that automatically functions to provide us with dissatisfied thoughts. This is why it was so easy to answer the second question. Instead, we need to stare directly at this context in action and observe it operating as it creates our dissatisfied thoughts.

When it comes to saving ourselves, we want to view that as our stubbornness to let go of this context. It is similar to when we struggle to apologize when we know we are wrong. Likewise, when another person mistakenly thinks we are unhappy and then asks about it, only to then force a negative feeling or complain to gain their sympathy. It is a choice to remain petty and frustrated with a situation even though it only makes things worse. The observer part in us is well aware that we are being irrational, yet we ignore that and return to listening to the dissatisfied thoughts until we feel frustrated. At this point, our thoughts seem logical and justified as our meaning-making machine creates more thoughts to explain the emotion. We want to catch ourselves doing this and stop it before it is too late. This is because, at the end of the day, the justifications for whatever negative emotion you are having has nothing to do with actually experiencing what you are after. So, while this might feel embarrassing to read and acknowledge as something we do, it is through observing this pettiness that we gain control over it.

Like anything, it is a skill set, but as you continue to do this, you will notice you spend more time enjoying yourself and less time trying to prevent pain. You will quit living your life in a way where you are afraid of wasting your good moods. This will enable you to stop needing reasons or rules to be met before you allow yourself happiness. You will start bringing satisfaction into situations that you previously felt justified to withhold it from. For example, a relationship you have some resentment towards for whatever reason or a job you perceived as a dead end.

While dissatisfaction may motivate you to change your circumstance, it is the satisfaction you bring that will change your life.

If you can allow yourself to show up and commit to just observing the content in your life for what it is and completely exist with it as it is - you will find things will start to show up as you wanted in the first place.

| WHY DO I HAVE NEVER-ENDING PROBLEMS? |

Humanity has come a long way. We have not only evolved out of a food chain but have found common languages to share thoughts and experiences. We have continued to advance our life expectancy as a species each year, as well as developing technology to connect and communicate with others on a mass scale. You would think that with all of our scientific advancements and thousands of years of profound philosophical wisdom that we would have figured out a perfect way to live. However, there has not been a perfect way to live that works for all people. Despite the fact that there are individuals who are able to manage their emotional needs, each individual is constantly at war with the way they are trying to meet those needs. Struggling with feelings of underwhelm and overwhelm that feed into the movies we believe we are in.

One of the reasons we stay dissatisfied in either overwhelm or underwhelm is because we are only ever managing paradoxical desires. Every single one of us is constantly battling a bunch of emotional needs that pull us in opposite directions. This forces us to live on one side or another of a spectrum of psychological desires. Take for example our need for community versus individuality. One part of us needs to feel connected and close to the people in our life. This comes out as an emotional need for love and comradery with our friends and family. Yet paradoxically, we also want to feel important and valued. This shows up as a desire to be better than others and rely on no one, where we can be completely free and independent in life.

These emotional needs for community and individuality are paradoxical, meaning they cannot both exist at the same time. So we are only ever living on one side of this paradox at any given moment. This is also why there is not one perfect way of being for everyone. Understanding this is one of the keys to realizing your life is not just a terrible movie with never-ending challenges. It is really just us misunderstanding that:

We all have paradoxical needs, not consistent problems.

Despite a belief that you might have never-ending challenges, you are really only fighting with yourself as you attempt to meet multiple emotional needs at the same time. This shows up as preferences and motivations that play out as movies we think we are living in.

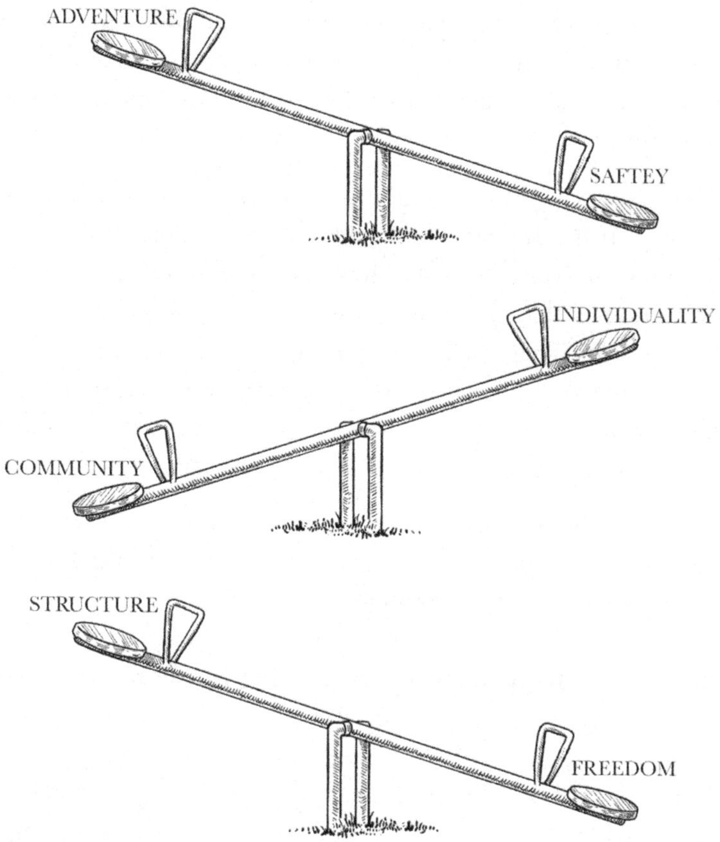

| EXISTENTIAL ISSUES |

A common experience people have when dismantling their movies is a feeling of emptiness. This comes from a realization that what was once motivating them is no longer important. For example, realizing that the promotion they thought would solve their dissatisfaction no longer motivates them. Or realizing that efforts of repeatedly arguing with their partner about the same issues is nothing more than time spent fighting about different values. Neither of these belong to a movie where they end up happy later.

This breakdown of the meaning that was once driving our behaviors is a good thing. It is a fresh canvas in which a new, more deliberate set of motivations can come through. However, a common misconception of this sensation is that this loss of meaning is a existential crisis or an existential issue. That label is nothing more than our mind's need to place meaning to experience. It is a description of a sensation that justifies another movie in which you solve the existential crisis and get to a place where all of your meaning is restored, and all is well.

As with all movies we make up, we never get to the good part. This trap of the existential issue is nothing more than a person over-entertaining their mind's ability to create thoughts. Observe this:

What actually happens to a person going through an existential crisis?

Nothing. There is nothing that is happening to that person other than the distressed look on their face. Their body is still just standing there unaffected and out of danger. Yet, it is their over-engagement with their mind's ability to create thought that causes this sensation. While it may seem too simplistic to dismiss, a person only needs to either:

1) Stop the act of thinking about thinking to have this existential issue vanish.

2) Overwhelm their mind with new behaviors and decisions so they have too much new stimulus to process.

3) Observe themselves creating the meaning of an existential issue.

When we do either of these, the mind returns to its automatic default of the need to make meaning, which forces us to re-indulge in the story of a movie. So, individuals who go through existential issues are actually doing something to themselves to get that effect. They are overthinking themselves into the corner of the room metaphorically, believing that their overthinking is productive to their happiness, when in actuality, it is just a person buying into yet another movie.

| WHY ME? |

A common experience of our thoughts "having us" is the meaning they place to why things happen to us. All of us, at some point or another, have interpreted a circumstance or situation as a personal attack on us, as in:

- “Of course I did not get the promotion - I never get what I deserve.”
- “They rejected ME even though I really liked them. Maybe I AM worthless.”
- “Someone damaged MY car, just one more thing for ME to deal with.”

This language, whether internal as a thought or external as a complaint, is nothing more than a flawed belief. It is a belief that the things that happen to us have objective meaning. As if those circumstances are all part of a movie in which we are repeatedly inconvenienced and disadvantaged for the sake of entertainment. You will know when people believe this because they also believe that their complaints matter. They believe that compulsively sharing their complaints and opinions can influence what has already happened and that by complaining to themselves and others, they can change what is. All of this follows the logic of it starting to rain outside just to make someone’s life harder, when in reality,

Life is not happening to you, but rather for you to experience.

Our life is an opportunity to experience what is. To have the chance to go through and interpret the world for enjoyment's sake. It is not a personal vendetta against us that we have to win or defeat; it is a space to explore and expand ourselves within. A collection of endless possibilities to live through and observe. Yet, when we complain to ourselves or others, we diminish this to a simple movie which cannot end well.

This is another one of those pills that is difficult to swallow because it is so second nature for us to complain or share our experiences. However, if you really want to see how much your opinion matters in the grand scheme of your life in this world, go share it with nature. Go tell nature what you think about politics or how you feel about what this or that person did. Go talk for hours with a tree about the gossip and drama at work or how your partner did not listen to you or care that one time. Try measuring how much change that actually makes to the quality of your life. While that seems dumb, what is even dumber is wasting both your time and someone else's with complaints. Because of this tendency to believe that life is out to get us and that our complaints can somehow change things, the majority of us get caught up in conversations that do not mean anything - like having a one-way conversation with a tree. When people approach conversations like this, they have little regard for the feedback of the other person. This results in us missing out on potential conversations that could be productive or meaningful. Ones where the context of the conversations is about connecting and relating to the other person, not just satisfying our compulsion to complain.

When you realize that your interactions and circumstances are just an opportunity to engage, you will free yourself from the previous mental movies that once limited you as a human being.

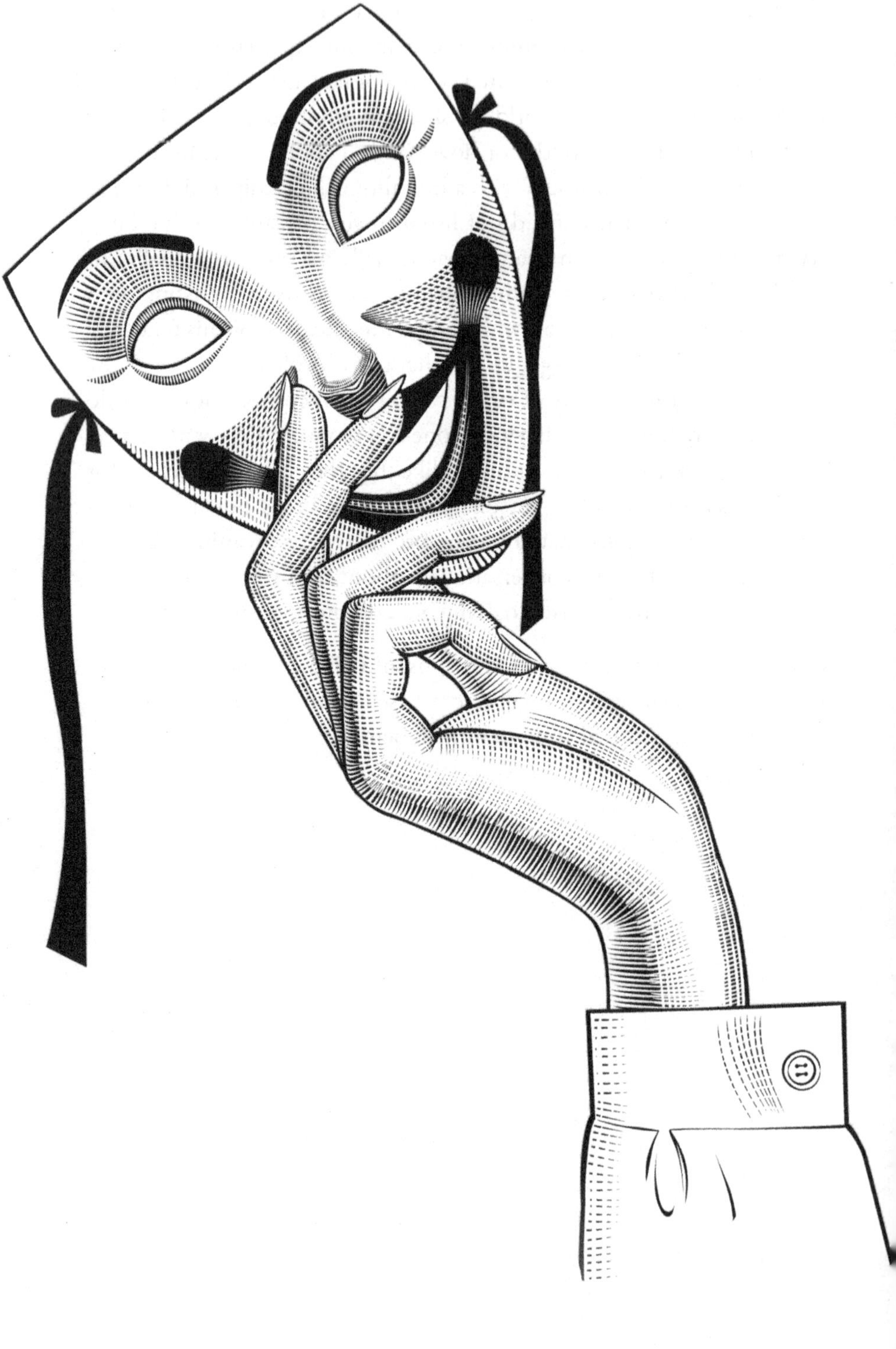

CHAPTER SIX

LOOKING GOOD

| SORTING OURSELVES |

Each and every person you look at is sorting themselves out. While they might appear confident and in control or carefree with a relaxed demeanor, everyone is working through some private personal issue. Issues like these often present themselves as things that other people seem to have already solved. These issues can include insecurities, fear, anger, compulsive lying, or impulsive behaviors, to name just a few. While there are many variations of these, the number and severity of them can vary depending on the individual. Yet, their common theme is one of shame and our desire to hide them. Regardless of your awareness of them, if you are human, you have them. They fuel a large portion of your motivations and identity with others. If it is not clear to you now, just answer this question:

What would you not want people to know about you?

If you just read past that without giving it an honest consideration, you are doing yourself a disservice by continuing without awareness of it. Your honest answer to that question is the driving force behind a large amount of your life. It is the harm we believe the snake will do to us if we confront it. So until we face it, we are stuck managing it privately and assuming no one else has these issues. While we imagine that these issues seem small to other people, they are huge to us - like a cut in our mouth that feels magnified. These issues seem to cause us to compulsively act, feel, and think in ways we cannot control, such as:

- Feeling worthless or inadequate
- Having low self-esteem or lacking confidence
- Struggling with a hot temper or repetitive anger
- Struggling to control a sexual impulse or thought
- Feeling shame about random violent or unusual imaginations
- Inability to forgive or let something go
- Feeling irrational or erratic emotions
- Feeling embarrassed about your inability to stop overthinking everything
- Feeling like you are still a child and unable to be an adult
- Having thoughts that you are secretly crazy
- Feeling lonely or unable to connect to people
- Feeling repetitively envious or petty towards others
- Having jealousy in a relationship
- Compulsively lying or misperceiving the truth
- Inability to be vulnerable or open up
- Fear of experiencing emotional or physical intimacy
- Feeling like you do not fit in or belong
- Fear of being abandoned or rejected
- Fear of failing or disappointing people
- Fear of public shame or embarrassment
- Having a need to control or change people
- Being unable to stand up for yourself or communicate your needs

- Feeling unattractive or undesired
- Having repetitive paranoia that everyone dislikes you
- Struggling to care or have more empathy for someone you should
- Feeling undeserving of love
- Feeling like your work is not good enough
- Feeling like you are never financially safe enough

While this is far from an exhaustive list, the common theme and belief we have about these reactions is:

"If people knew the real me, they would not like me."

While the origin of this belief is only a subjective interpretation, given the logic of our exploration into ourselves thus far, we can assume this came about in some variation of the fact we are wired for survival. As infants and children, our survival relied solely on the people who raised us. Meaning that their approval, love, and care was a matter of life or death to our younger selves. At some point in our childhood, we experience a loss of approval, love, or care that we, from this young age, interpret as a trauma. Regardless of the quality of our upbringing, all children experience this when we first have our careless curiosity and exploration of the world suddenly stopped by an adult trying to keep us safe. It could have been by running out on a busy road, misbehaving with our parents in a store, or attempting to touch a hot stove. Either way, the moment we first experience a parent yell, shame, guilt, or correcting us, our young brains interpret that experience as the withdrawal of love and care. From that point, it is safe to assume that our young mind concludes some variation of:

"Love and care are conditional, which means my survival relies on meeting conditions."

As a result, our minds begin to perceive that we are unworthy of love and care or that we will lose love and care if we fail. Both of which trigger compulsive thoughts and behaviors as a way to avoid this perceived truth. These patterns then develop into a personality and identity which justify this avoidance in the form of the insecurities and issues we mentioned initially.

CHILDHOOD CONCLUSION THAT "**LOVE AND CARE ARE CONDITIONAL**"

ASSUMPTION THAT "**I'M UNWORTHY OF LOVE / IF I FAIL I WON'T BE LOVED**"

ATTEMPTS TO AVOID THIS BELIEF WITH **COMPULSIVE BEHAVIORS & DEFENSIVE THOUGHTS**

INTRODUCTION OF **INSECURITY & UNNECESSARY ISSUES**

FORMATION OF A **PERSONALITY & IDENTITY TO JUSTIFY PROBLEMS**

If this at all feels unrelated to you or you are unaware of how this is affecting your life today, just answer these questions:

As a child, whose love and attention did you crave and want most growing up? Your mom, dad, grandparent, relative or guardian?

When you have identified the person, ask yourself:

Who did you have to be for them in order to get their approval?

Your answers to this question are likely a description of the current identity and personality traits you compulsively live out now in an effort to avoid the snake. While it can feel embarrassing to admit to ourselves, let alone other people, these fears and the insecurities that protect us influence:

- The rules we force ourselves to follow
- The opportunities we justify avoiding
- The excuses we give into
- The stories we tell ourselves about others
- The assumptions we make about the world
- The generalizations about the world
- The unhealthy narratives we subscribe to
- The beliefs we hold about what is possible
- The limitations we place on others
- The logic and reasoning we insist are correct
- The best practices we follow
- The self-sabotaging behaviors we engage in
- The arguments we have to win
- The need to be right or get our way
- The past baggage we refuse to let go

- The toxic relationships we keep ignoring
- The addictions we maintain and think we control
- The avoidance of rejection
- The obsessive desire to feel validated
- The achievements we want others to believe we have
- The roles and responsibilities we take
- The grudges we hold onto
- The compulsive behaviors that harm us
- The rationalizations we tell ourselves about our unethical behavior
- The lies and exaggerations we tell other people and ourselves
- The image or public opinion we maintain
- The radically irrational avoidance of being judged or embarrassed
- The pettiness we hold over others who have made mistakes
- The advice we give to others that we do not follow
- The many things we do that do not help us

Again, this is far from a complete list but it is long enough for you to understand that we all have many strategies for avoiding the snake, most of which we compulsively attempt to hide from ourselves and other people. Part of the reason for this is their seemingly simple and small nature of them. If we are aware of them, we tend to beat ourselves up for not having it handled. Worst of all, it appears through our observation and interactions with other people that they do not have our issues. So even if we were to solve them, they would not merit any public praise because it is expected that they should not exist in the first place. That makes these issues and insecurities carry a lot of shame around them. Thus, we have the desire to try to ignore them or present ourselves as people who do not have them. But regardless of our efforts, they come out and control our lives if we do not face them. It is helpful to understand that:

The more personal the issue, the more universal the issue.

The issues that cause you the most pain and fear in your life are also the most common. Regardless of your belief that it must be only you going through them, to be human is to have these fears and insecurities. But it is in our un-acknowledgment and avoidance of them that we waste our lives.

We do this by spending our time on earth trying to look good and trying to make our movies come true, attempting to give off the impression that we are not having any issues and insecurities. We try to look like we have it all figured out and that our lives work. When in actuality, you, me, and everyone else are only ever making it up as we go.

Now, this should not be suggesting you run off and spend your life in therapy. Rather, it is just an invitation to be authentic about our inauthentic tendencies. As soon as we do this, we can start to handle the things that previously handled us.

THE MORE PERSONAL THE ISSUE,
THE MORE UNIVERSAL THE ISSUE.

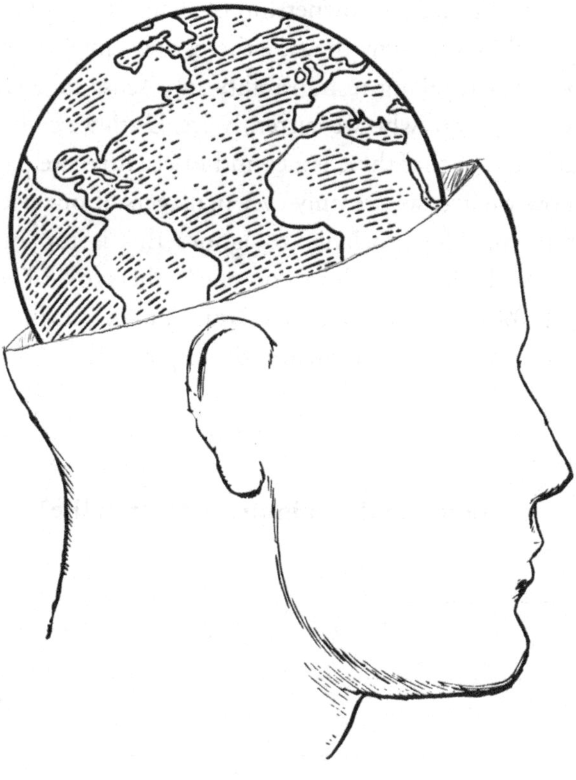

| RESPONSIBILITY |

So, where does personal responsibility come into all of this? Well as we explored in part one, in order for us to observe something, we need to know what it is and what our role in it is. Regardless of why our insecurities and issues are present or who is to blame or at fault for the circumstances, we believe and justify them. If we want any hope of being able to stand our ground with these problematic qualities in ourselves, we must first take ownership of them. This is not necessarily taking responsibility for why they are there, as we might not have had a say in that. Rather, taking responsibility in a sense of ownership that these traits are a part of who we currently are. Until we come face to face with this and accept that these issues and insecurities are part of us and influence how we live, we are only ever managers of our lives and never owners of them. The proclivity to ignore this is too easy and too habitual for us which is why almost no one bothers to deal with it. Until we manage 100% of us as we are, those issues and insecurities manage us. So, take some time to seriously answer these questions:

Where could you improve most in life?

___

___

___

___

What has stopped you from doing that?

Now attach the word 'because' to the end of your answers and finish the statements in a way that places the responsibility on you for that outcome. Word your answers in a way that demonstrates how you do not let, give, or make something possible. Do not worry about accuracy, just aim for potency. See some examples below:

- People do not support me **because I am unsupportable.**
- My partner does not really want me **because I do not let myself be wanted.**
- I do not have enough time **because I do not make the time to do it.**
- I am unable to do that **because I do not make myself able.**
- The marketplace does not want my product **because I do not give what the marketplace wants.**
- There are not enough customers **because I do not give enough to customers.**
- My partner does not care about fixing us **because I do not let myself be fixed.**

Simply add the word "because" to the end of your reasons from the previous page and complete the sentence in a way that holds you accountable for the outcome. Again, this isn't about being accurate or correct. The point of this is to break the mental habits of seeing our challenges in a certain light.

While we are just playing with language, our goal is to take responsibility through ownership. Again, not for how this situation or issue came to be. Rather it's about taking ownership of where it goes from here and taking responsibility for the experience those issues and insecurities cause moving forward.

After doing this, you might feel like the next step is to try and solve this new statement by changing the circumstance of it. However, that is not our goal. What we need is not new circumstances to paint with context, but rather to stop painting. Right now, we only need to observe and become aware of what we do to ourselves with these meanings. This will enable us to experience our circumstances without meaning, just as it is without it being part of a movie.

It is only from a place of seeing life without paint that we can have any say in what color goes on next. You cannot jump from one movie to another without leaving the theater first meaning:

You need to first realize *who* you really are before you can have any say in *how* you are.

Start to own and stand with what used to own you. Really allow yourself to accept your issues and insecurities for what they are. Just your particular struggles. Once you accept them as just a part of you, they lose any power they had over you. This is the real first step to overcoming our insecurities.

| LIFE IS SO COMPLICATED |

Be it our dating lives, careers, or personal way of life, simplicity is not our strong suit. This is not because we make our lives complicated, instead, complication happens when we do not simplify them. Having a complicated life is the default reaction of living a life without examining it. Take into account all of the mechanisms and mental processes we have explored so far. If left unexamined, they lock us into complex lives, full of rules in the form of have-tos and "if this happens, then that". Making, everything we do in our life require justification and thought-out reasoning, beyond enjoyment alone. The more concerning element is the complexity found in our interactions with other people. We start off with good intentions, picking partners from a place of enjoyment. However, many people end up staying in relationships because of previous feelings that do not resemble present experiences. We cling onto a promise of how a relationship could be, although it has not been that way since the beginning. Or take for example a job we dislike or a business that is dysfunctional. We keep doing things we hate because we think the financial outcomes can in some way make up for our initial dissatisfaction. Our life ends up being a multitude of different rules and justifications to satisfy our survival proclivity to maximize pleasure and minimize the effort required to do so.

One of the more complicated areas of our life comes down to our identity. We complicate our lives because our identities are rewarded. This means we self-create obstacles and problems so that our identities can remain valid and useful. Take for example what you believe your friends like about you. More often than not, we will find ways to maintain those qualities even if it makes our lives harder.

Answer this:

What do you think your friends enjoy most about you?

If we take that answer and look at that quality, we can see that it relies on a problem existing within your life or in other people's lives. The same way a religious skeptic needs a church. We tend to complicate our lives with the addition of problems so that our identities and ways of being admired can exist.

If you believe that you are loved for your ability to solve problems, you need problems to be loved. If you believe that your kindness is what your friends love most about you, then you need to be surrounded by unkindness to be loved. If it is because you are fun, then you need to be with unfun people to feel loved. If it is all the drama you go through, then you need to have drama to be loved.

Not all traits in us are bad. The goal is not to demonize our positive qualities, but just to keep an eye on how those qualities are maintained in our life. This is important because our need for admiration and validation will almost always trump our desire for happiness. This means, more often than not:

You would rather feel validated than happy.

The dopamine we experience when we are right and confirm our way of being is incredibly addictive, more so than when we use introspection to simplify our lives. This is why more people choose to complicate their life and self-sabotage their happiness than work through their need for validation.

Take a moment now to examine these questions for yourself.

Are you purposely creating problems or surrounding yourself in unproductive company?

Does your identity rely on the validation of others?

Are there qualities in yourself that keep you away from peace and contentment?

Where are you unnecessarily complicating your life?

By taking the time to ask yourself questions like these, you can start to simplify your life, thus creating space for a more deliberate and proactive life.

| INCONGRUENCE |

Have you ever had the experience of ease or flow with a goal you wanted to accomplish? As a whole, the entire process, from the beginning as a thought to its completion as an action, seemed effortless. Almost as though you were pulled through it by your mind and body instead of having to push yourself and use willpower. While this could have been a challenging or simple task, there was a feeling of inner alignment in your thoughts, words, and actions. As a result of the clarity you had around pursuing this desire, motivation did not even register as a need. Sometimes, it is the creative inspiration we get for a project, and other times, it is our impulse to clean our room or car as a procrastination tactic. Either way, the transition from just a thought to something tangible or completed happened seamlessly.

This alignment of what we believe we can do, what we intend to do, and what we actually do is what we call congruence.

While it tends to just be a random experience for most of us, there is a recipe for how a person gets into that state - an awareness of the inner clarifications needed to produce this experience.

As explained in the previous section, we complicate our lives. One of the ways this complication happens is when we do not take the time to clarify and align our beliefs, intentions, and actions.

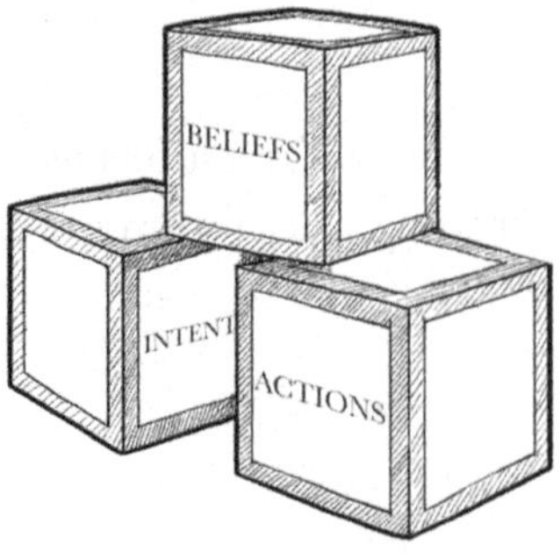

When these three things do not add up, we live in a state of incongruence. Here is an example of what this looks like: say someone wants to write a book, so they have the intention of writing one. They also believe they have a compelling story and the ability to write it well. Despite these two factors, they do not take action. They talk a lot about it and spend a lot of time in their head thinking about it, but they do not spend any time writing it. Instead, they just tell everyone about it, saying how they should or could do it. That's one form of incongruence.

Another example could be someone who has the intention of keeping their weight under control. With their intention clear, they even manage to take action towards it by going to the gym and attempting to eat well. Yet they struggle to keep the weight off once they lose it, constantly falling back into their previous unhealthy habits. This is because their beliefs are off about who they are. In this case, there is not an inner version of themself that is aligned with being able to maintain their weight. So, the incongruence of their beliefs keeps them frustrated with a fluctuation in their weight.

A common example of this can be had if you imagine yourself as you are, driving up to a red light on a road. Rolling up next to you is your dream car in the exact color you want. As the window rolls down, you see someone who's the same gender and age as you. Without any distinct or defining look on their face, they continue to drive up the road as the light turns green. As you imagine this, I want you to think about who that person is.

What are the thoughts that instantly popped into your head about who that person might be?

What are the first things that come to mind?
What do you think about who they are?
What are they like?
How could they afford that car?
What's their story?
What attributes do you think their personality has?

You might find that the initial answers that came to your mind were along the lines of:

- They are spoiled or greedy
- They came from a rich family
- They are probably a snob or arrogant
- They are not in touch with reality
- Any variation of the above

If you found that your answers were negative, you have an incongruence towards getting that car. The problem a lot of people face is that even though they might want that car, they cannot become something they hate. So, if you think the only way to acquire a car like that is to come from an affluent family or be greedy or manipulative, it is impossible for you to actually obtain that.

You cannot become something you hate or you become the hate.

This statement really demonstrates part of the way we complicate our lives. On the one hand, we need to make sense of why we do not have what we want so we create stories that justify and excuse our circumstances. Yet, we also allow ourselves to desire those outcomes and create movies about getting them. This incongruence makes us hesitant, half-hearted, and uncommitted toward life, never letting us fully sink our teeth into situations and opportunities. As explained before, we care more about saving ourselves, looking good, being right, and defending our way of being. This means we almost never allow ourselves to give our all into what we do for fear of failure, embarrassment, or confirming our insecurities. As a result, we continue living in ways that keep us where we are instead of genuinely progressing forward into situations that are more enjoyable. We make our life about looking good rather than feeling good, which is something we tend to have a lot of congruence with.

So as you think to yourself, or interact with others, ask yourself:

What are my beliefs around achieving what I want?

Am I willing to let go of negative justifications for my lack of results in order to obtain them?

Would I rather be right or happy right now?

| JUSTIFICATION |

Another way we complicate our life is by using our justifications to keep us in situations that can never match our ideal circumstance. Such as staying in a job or relationship that is "just good" but not great. While simultaneously believing that we could get something great while still holding onto what we believe is "just good". This logic looks a lot like:

- “While I like my partner for where I am in life, I know that if I was more successful, I would not be with them”.

This logic justifies keeping a relationship that would not exist should a more successful version of us also exist. The issue with this logic is that it does not account for how our mental movies keep success or happiness in the distant future. So, because our mind creates stories based on our current circumstance, the successful version of ourselves could never occur alongside the circumstance of our current relationship. Meaning by choosing to stay in that relationship you would also simultaneously be choosing the unsuccessful version of yourself. It is this type of logic that complicates our lives and keeps us trapped in situations for years that never make us happy - be it a relationship or job. Part of where this logic comes from is our obsession to maximize the reduction of pain and the gaining of pleasure, while minimizing the effort required in doing that.

This process of justification complicates our life by never allowing us to make space for better situations to occur. It keeps us holding on to situations that simultaneously make it impossible to get what we are after, as a result of our own logic.

Keep in mind, that this is not a suggestion that you just quit your job, end your relationship, or make drastic changes to your circumstances in life if they are making you unhappy. Again, this is just about exposing the ways in which we complicate our lives and make ourselves unhappy. From seeing just how we make happiness and satisfaction impossible, we can then accurately observe our circumstances for how they fit into what makes us happy. This means that after we clear away all the movies and rules, if they no longer make sense to keep, then it is worth letting go. This is about simplifying our lives by exposing unnecessary complications or by deconstructing circumstances for what they actually are. So, let's take a moment to identify where these justifications can be holding you back.

Think about a satisfied and successful version of yourself.

Now, without trying to manipulate the image, answer these questions honestly:

Does your current job, relationship, or circumstance, as it is right now, exist in that vision?

Without changing anything about how you are currently experiencing your life, what parts of it remain in your ideal self?

Your answers will help you identify any unintentional limitations you have placed on yourself.

CHAPTER SEVEN

WHY YOU DO WHAT YOU DO

| BEHIND MOTIVATION |

As part of our desire to improve, we also paradoxically do not want to change. Going back to our biological need for safety, we addictively hold onto our habits of survival while also psychologically pushing for new outcomes. This creates an internal tug of war with ourselves.

This tug of war is very obvious when we shine a light on why we want most things. Say you want the motivation to lose weight, start a business, or create music. The problem for most people is found when they actually dive into why they are motivated. As we explored earlier, when a person continually asks "why?" they will notice it more often stems from an insecurity or assumption of scarcity.

Here is a typical internal dialogue for example:

> "Why do you want to lose weight?"
> "Because I want to be skinny"
> "Why?"
> "Because I want to look good"
> "Why?"
> "Because I want to be attractive"
> "Why?"
> "Because I want to get into a relationship"
> "Why?"
> "Because I do not want to be lonely"
> "Why?"
> "Because I want to be loved"
> "Why?"
> "Because if I'm not loved I feel bad"
> "Why?"
> "Because it confirms the assumption that I'm afraid that I'm not worthy of love."

If we ask why we want something over and over, we will uncover a part of ourselves that is often petty, insecure, selfish, or some other unpleasant trait.

However, it is important to remember that those thoughts are only conclusions that show up because of our biological wiring. Just like with our snake, neither is accurate - both are by-products of a survival-based context in which these types of thoughts appear. After that, our ego rationalizes and defends the actions and decisions we take to avoid those thoughts. So, to really acknowledge this primal motive in ourselves requires the courage to turn a light on these dark elements of our nature with determined self-inquiry. This is why we have continually asked questions throughout this book. Until we answer them, we continue to allow our source of motivation to come from a scarcity-based, biological nature that is just trying to avoid pain. The issue with this is that:

Any action made from a place of scarcity can only ever reinforce the place it came from.

So, if you are losing weight because you want to solve your insecurity, you will only ever increase the insecurity you feel, regardless of the weight loss. Alternatively, if your motivation to lose weight came from a context of loving yourself, you would simultaneously release the insecurity and be naturally motivated to lose weight. Every action taken from that context would produce thoughts that honor and uplift you, rather than thoughts that only minimize your insecurity but never remove it.

| A NEED TO ACHIEVE |

This business of changing context is important when we look at our motivations. Regardless of our results and drive, our efforts are meaningless if they are from the wrong context. Just as we explained in part one, we live as though we are avoiding a snake. Therefore, any action taken to avoid the snake only ever keeps the snake in the corner, never really addressing the issue of the snake itself. Analogy aside, keep the following statements in mind:

Any achievement made from trying to not be a failure can never remove the fear you have of being a failure – it can only push it away.

Any relationship you get from a place of trying to be happy will never solve the unhappiness - it can only temporarily distract you from it.

Any job or title you get to prove your worth can never fix your feeling of worthlessness – it can only suspend it.

The problem with this is that:

No external circumstance can truly heal, nourish, or satiate an internal condition.

What we need is an internal solution for an internal issue. Although a change of external circumstance may feel different, it is only temporary, until the underlying internal issue surfaces as a new problem, hurdle, or inconvenience in our life. It is like trying to bail the water out of a boat with holes in it. Our imagination can consistently create problems as easily as it can create excuses for what we do not want to do. Making the chase for external solutions never-ending.

Additionally, as long as you keep using an external band-aid to try and fix an internal wound, you keep the solution separate and detached from you. This means you can always lose it or have it taken away from you. This is why we get protective, defensive, and attached to these external strategies and circumstances. Anything that we cannot solve internally means we are always being externally controlled by it, like an addiction we no longer have a choice in. When we cannot self-create the emotions we need, we will always rely on other people, things, and situations to do it for us. This can look like:

- A compulsive need for money when what you really need is the internal emotion of security

- An insatiable desire for attention or sex when what you really need is the internal feeling of love

- An overwhelming pressure to achieve when what you really need is an internal realization of worthiness

Almost all of our wants, desires, needs, and must-haves can be obtained internally when we understand what emotion we are really after - with the only exclusions being our biological needs like food, water, and physical safety. While this might seem inaccurate to read at first, all you have to do is peel back the curtains on why you want what you want. From here, you will be able to see the underlying internal emotion you believe that external thing will give you.

We do not actually want the sports car, mansion, or supermodel. We want the emotions we believe those things will give us.

At the heart of all achievement, behavior, or desire, we ultimately want emotion. What we are really after is not an external circumstance, but rather an internal condition. Our confusion in this comes from how we allow ourselves to feel these emotions when we get these things. The process of internally feeling negative then having something external happen and internally feeling positive seems seamless. But in reality, it only appears seamless because we have become so skilled at repeating this process. From the first time we concluded that love is conditional and felt the withdrawal of it, we have chased external circumstances to satisfy internal desires. Even though this was a fair and logical interpretation for our young minds to make at that time. It is clearly inaccurate, when observed with our more developed minds as adults. Returning to our interpretation of the internal condition being attached to the external circumstance, it is important to remember that these things are actually separate and unattached - it is us who attaches them. In the absence of human beings, the world is meaningless, emotionless, and devoid of any rules regarding when internal conditions should appear. All of the external circumstances just exist separately as they are without meaning. It is through our internal allowing of positive emotions that we create our sensations of pleasure. The external circumstances are only the rules we keep as to when we think it is internally appropriate.

If you are still skeptical of this, imagine that you have just received a random phone call from an attorney. This lawyer has been in charge of a will set out by an old acquaintance. For whatever reason, they have placed you as the sole inheritor of their large family fortune which is worth multiple millions. As they confirm who you are and start to lay out the process of how this money unfolds into your life, you feel the skepticism start to fade. This then makes this situation seem very real as a sense of excitement and possibility enters your mind. You start to see how your stress and worry about the future will disappear. Your mind bursts with creativity as you think of a variety of new ways you will enjoy yourself. As the conversation ends after collecting the details, you are left right where you once were before you picked up the call, yet in a completely different experience. Nothing has changed about your external circumstances or you physically. No money has been deposited into your account yet. It is still just you in your head, only with a completely different internal condition. It was only by your allowance of a new internal condition that you felt this way. In theory, you could have still accessed that same level of excitement or that same security about your future without that phone call. But, due to our habit of looking externally, this internal solution seems inappropriate. This comes from our comfort of using dissatisfaction and negative emotion to push us into new circumstances. Yet, as we explored previously, any action taken from that place can never truly solve what we are ultimately after, which is an internal condition of happiness and contentment.

Similarly, if moments after the call ended, the attorney called you back only to tell you a mistake was made and to apologize for the confusion as you would no longer inherit anything, you would still do this process. However, this time you would just create a new internal condition that contained thoughts of scarcity, limitation, and fear. You have still had nothing change about your external circumstances other than the time that passed to experience all of this.

So, while external circumstances can sometimes feel more direct in their influence on our emotions than our ability to just create new internal conditions, what is important is to understand the role we play in how our experience unfolds. That awareness is what allows us more control over our life, regardless of how potent external circumstances can be.

| GOING IN TO GET OUT |

Another reason why we need to solve our internal issues first is because of how they inadvertently cause new external circumstances to show up. Our goal is not to trim each external leaf one by one in our life so that we no longer feel their internal reactions. Instead, it is to examine the internal roots of these issues so that we can get to the foundations of why certain external circumstances continue to show up in our life.

Take for example the experience of repeatedly attracting unhealthy or toxic relationships. To assume you randomly encounter these partners would be inaccurate. There are actually many factors, both known and also unknown, that are dictating your attraction to these people. While it can be a lifelong task to fully understand these external factors for many social scientists and PhDs, you only need to understand the internal root causes that produce the external circumstances to gain control over them. But to demonstrate this, we can look at the difference of effort required to solve this both externally and internally.

Let's start by diving into the complexity of the understanding needed to create an external solution.

- Imagine a depressed person. Immediately, you might have an image of their slouched posture, shallow breathing, and defeated face. Alternatively, if you were to imagine a confident person, you might visualize someone with a strong upright posture, full breath, and a focused or smiling face. You are able to do this because almost all humans are wired to be practical psychologists. This means that they are able to pick up on social cues and are hypersensitive to body language. Odds are you could even tell the emotions of a complete stranger passing by with just a few glances.

- Now let's look at another factor. Imagine for example that you only ever worked out your right arm in the gym. For weeks and even months, you would only do bicep curls only with your right arm. Eventually, you would be able to visibly see the difference between your left and right arm. So, if we know that there is a physical look to someone who is feeling depressed or confident, we can also assume that a person who repeatedly feels a certain emotion will hold their body in the physiology that matches that emotion. Through consistent repetition, they will also start to build a muscular contortion towards the physiology of that emotion. Even if it is only shown slightly, this would be easy for our mind's hypersensitivity to body language to spot.

- If you have struggled to find a healthy relationship and you are repeatedly in an emotional state of sadness and neediness, there is a good chance you are also unconsciously communicating to other people that you are going to make them sad. Then that neediness will also come out through additional insecure behavior. Inadvertently causing you more of what you have already experienced in your life.

- In the case of bad relationships that repeatedly trigger painful flashbacks, there's a good chance you're unconsciously communicating to others that you are familiar with being treated badly. This inadvertently invites people with patterns of treating their partners poorly. In turn, this produces more relationships similar to what you have already experienced.

While these are just assumptions, we can also imagine that there are many other external factors like this happening in the background as well. Nevertheless, this is important in our external example to demonstrate how many complex understandings are required in order to control this outcome of repeated toxic relationships.

Instead, we can dive right to the root of the issue by understanding the role our internal conditions have on all of our experiences. Take for example if you had no understanding of any possible psychological explanations for what causes repeated toxic relationships. By simply solving the emotional internal condition, you would simultaneously solve all of the possible external solutions that could follow those understandings. This is achieved by first allowing yourself to feel happy, attractive, and respected without needing those emotions to come from an external partner. You would start to shift your physiology. If you did this repeatedly, you would create a muscular contortion that communicated those emotions to other people. After a short while, you would find that people would start to pay more positive attention to you because we are externally wearing our internal states. These are then picked up, either consciously or unconsciously, by other people, thereby helping you attract a better external environment.

When we talk about trying to control external factors as an effort to improve our lives, in our prior example, it would be like trying to fake your body language and communication all day long. And this would all be in an effort to trick every new person who randomly glances in your direction. As well as managing every other external factor that attracts people to you. This could range from things like pheromones, the environment, or anything else we are unaware of. Needless to say, it is not very practical, let alone possible. Rather, our best bet at solving our issues is by first solving the internal root of the issue, which are our internal conditions. We can do this by proactively using our mind's vivid memories and imagination. As an alternative to compulsively searching for an external solution, we can effectively use our internal ability of imagination to envision relationships that are better and healthier. We can also use our vivid memory to remember positive qualities and preferences we desire. Rather than focusing on the pains we experienced, we can focus on shifting our physiologies as well as the other numerous external factors that cause us to attract the people we do. This is why it is not only practical to start internally but it is also the necessary approach to solving our issues.

PART III

LIVING & ACTION

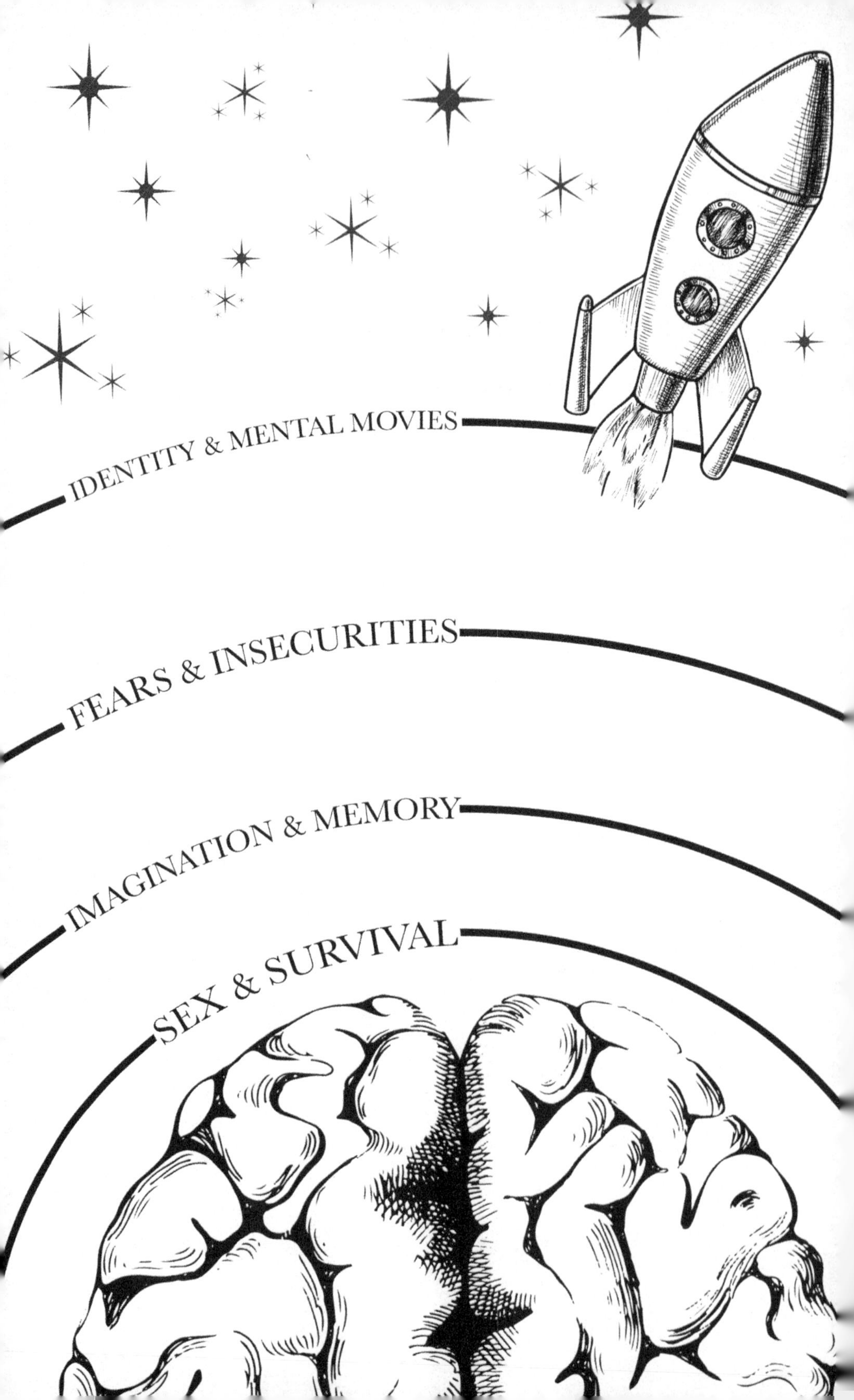
IDENTITY & MENTAL MOVIES
FEARS & INSECURITIES
IMAGINATION & MEMORY
SEX & SURVIVAL

CHAPTER EIGHT

PROCESS

| LAUNCHING INTO SPACE |

Imagine a spaceship launching itself into space, passing through the many layers of the earth's atmosphere. Going higher and further up into the sky until it gets far enough to be free from the pull of gravity that keeps us grounded to the earth. Once out in space, the ship almost appears weightless now that it is no longer limited and restricted by earth's natural forces. Now allowing it to float and move about with more ease as it completes a mission.

This is a lot like how a mind goes through awareness. Without it, we are restricted by the many natural forces that influence our lives like our biological need for sex and survival. Or our mind's obsession with creating mental movies to protect us from imagined snakes. However, as we observe these influences and gain awareness of them, we tend to break past a mental atmosphere. A place that is free from the pressure and struggles of underwhelm or overwhelm we previously experienced.

We are now able to navigate with minimal force as we no longer get in our own way. This awareness is like being weightless in that we are no longer weighed down by what previously held us back in life, now letting go of disempowering stories and fears. We can easily propel ourselves towards what we are really after, our ultimate purpose, which is happiness and contentment in life.

From this place, there is a lightness in our experience, be it personally, romantically, socially, or professionally. People who get here still have challenges and aspirations. However they experience them from a more proactive and willing place, no longer controlled by their insecurities or fears. Again, while they may still have issues, their issues do not *have* them. Instead, they experience problems from a distant view, like an astronaut floating in space and looking down on earth. This level of awareness allows us to not only detach from the painful compulsions and impulses of our mind and body but also to approach life more deliberately. Where we can experience our life as it is as well as from a more proactive context. One that uses our mind's tendencies as tools to fix what we can in life while featuring what we cannot change about ourselves and our circumstances.

In the last part of this book, we will finally apply what we have learned. We will approach every important aspect in our life from a place of awareness for what it is rather than what we imagine it as. We will observe the different parts of our life as though they were suspended in the vacuum of space, separated from the contexts that once limited it back on earth. From here, we can experience a new way to relate to ourselves, others, and the world.

| THE FEELING OF OBSERVATION |

We want to keep our spaceship analogy in mind. Just as you could imagine yourself as an astronaut floating weightlessly out in space, observing earth without being in it. We want to observe the important parts of our life as though they are suspended in space, without having to live with the pressure and weight of them. So, imagine our relationship, work, or a particular mental movie floating beside us, yet not giving us a sensation with its meaning. This feels a lot like acknowledging something is there, but not accepting it as anything more than something that we can point to. It is being able to play with an idea or sit with a belief without having to accept it as true or prove it wrong. It is just floating alongside something in space. We can allow it to exist as it is without trying to control, remove, or change it.

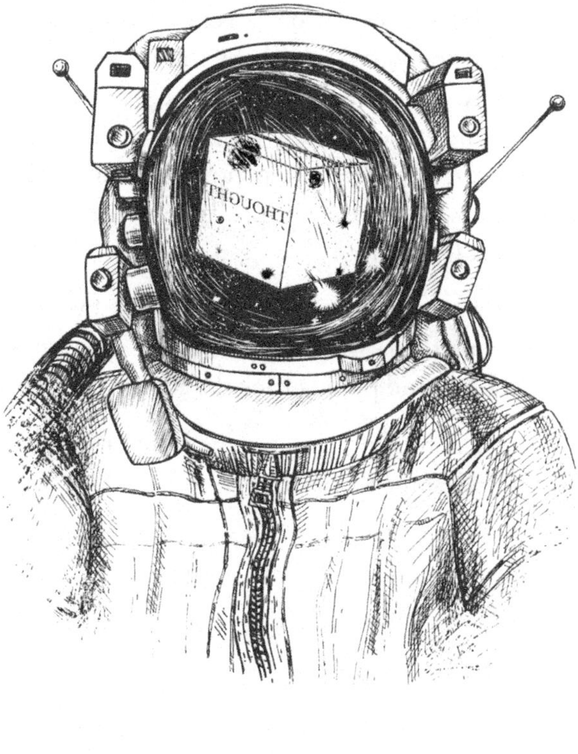

This experience is what we earlier described as observation. It is the internal act of reducing and dissecting the different parts of our mind as it perceives our circumstances. Again, this is not watching something to see if we agree or disagree with it or trying to study it in a way to predict and control it. It is simpler than that. It is just pointing to the thoughts that show up in your mind without trying to describe it with another thought, rather just experience it for what it is, while knowing where it came from. So, as you continue to read, fully sit with and entertain these ideas alongside you rather than trying to categorize them as right or accurate. Feel the concepts or claims on the following pages as experiences for you to entertain the possibility of, instead of something you need to like or prove wrong.

If you can do this, you can observe your life without context. As if looking at the contents of your life without the paint from a bucket of pre-decided context. While this is not a natural state for us to remain in, it is a natural thing for us to do and use as a tool. It is the act that allows us to deconstruct meaning and see things for what they are, as they are. Until we can do this, we cannot truly select a new context to experience our circumstances through. Which is why this is the first step in having any actual say in how life is experienced. So, we want to observe how we actually relate to life which means how we actually experience our relationships and circumstances. It is how we really spend our time when relating and what is really happening in the observable world instead of being just in our head.

One of the easiest ways to start doing this is by asking yourself questions. More particularly, use a style of questioning that is committed to exposing and pulling back the curtain on yourself.

As you find yourself thinking about something or caught up in your thoughts, ask yourself some variation of:

"How do I know this thought to be 100% true?"

"How does this actually relate to my happiness?"

"Does thinking this give me emotions I enjoy?"

"What part of me needs this to be accurate?"

"Are my meanings, assessments, and judgments just coming from my mood?"

"Why am I attached to this?"

"Why do I think this?"

Questions like these repeatedly asked to yourself will start to unveil the mechanisms we have explored in this book. As you start to do this, you will be able to return to yourself as an observer that is free from context. It takes practice like all skills. However, as you repeatedly do this throughout your life, you get quicker and quicker at it. You also get better at catching yourself engaging in unproductive contexts you did not decide on. This ultimately leads us to the ability to willfully re-engage with context.

| RETURNING TO EARTH |

Like the astronaut who returns back from a successful mission, we can willfully return back to the weight and pressure that comes from our minds placing meaning - the key word being *willfully*. Until you know you can break free from context, your problems and issues in life are still problems and issues. It is only once you can fully distance yourself through observation that you have any say in the way a situation shows up in your life. This is not about reframing our issues with positive thinking or ignorantly sticking our heads in the sand with denial. This is intellectually exposing *what is* versus *what is not* in life and breaking down how much of our time and effort is being wasted on *what is not*. When you have the ability to observe your life for what it actually is, you free yourself from the pressurized atmosphere that your mind creates. It is that ability that then allows you to contextualize your life from a place of choice. This is where you willfully take on those same problems and issues, only this time they show up as the *experience* of a challenge or opportunity to learn from. One last time for clarity, this is not about *thinking* of your problems as opportunities, as that is not emotionally real to us. If you do that, you are only lying to yourself about how it feels, hoping to change what is, making it another thing for you to mentally do. It is like an endless need to force gratitude without ever questioning why you are not grateful to begin with. If you are having this experience, you need to question yourself more. I would recommend rereading parts one and two to see how that type of thinking is not even yours and leads nowhere. This is not to say that you need to have the act of observation mastered; it is only that you should emotionally understand it and intellectually grasp it.

Having reached a place of being able to point to the ability of observation, this book now explores this awareness when applied to the most significant areas of life. But before that, it is important to consider the philosophical consequences and conclusions of this. Given that this is how you, me, and everyone else operates in life.

| THE DRY PHILOSOPHY OF IT ALL |

If observation is a choice and there is an ability in how we experience the world then we need to explore the ramifications of each option. On one side, we live in a suspended, detached state of observation. On the other, a submerged and engaged context that keeps us in overwhelm or underwhelm.

With both of these options available to us we are also presented with some philosophical dilemmas to work through. While these next few paragraphs are here to be read, it is not necessary to have a complete philosophical understanding to grasp the remainder of this book. Whatever the case may be, just continue reading on.

To start, we can conclude that we are both "whole in experience" yet "imperfect in thinking".

When we observe life as it is, the experience is "whole", in that it needs for nothing. Meaning life without context is both vivid and complete. Allowing us to experience it from a fully engaged space, in which we lose track of time and identities. It is when we get out of our heads and fully engage with a situation as it is, that we require nothing external from us. When this happens, we can conclude that experience by itself needs for nothing. It is complete and whole in nature.

It is through the engagement of our minds that we spot what is lacking and missing. Which pushes us to improve and desire new experiences in life. But the act of thinking is ultimately flawed in that our mental movies don't naturally lead us to happiness. Making these thoughts and mental movies unfinished and "imperfect" by nature.

It is when people confuse their thinking as "perfect" and experiences as "incomplete" that they waste their time in life. This results in never getting what they want as they are caught up in trying to make *what is* (content) *what it is not* (context). Rather, it is through seeing our relationships, work, and personal life through this idea of "whole yet imperfect" that we can make conclusions about how we should operate. If we approach our life as though it is whole and needs for nothing, we can let go of our attachment to our thoughts as valid needs. So, we start to approach our work and relationships without expectations or needs for them to be different. Taking on life from a place of already being satisfied.

We can go into the experience of our relationships and work looking to give more, instead of looking for what we can get out of them.

If this is all still sounding theoretical to you, that is alright. This is really just the philosophical explanation of what we have explored so you can be aware of the logic we are using in our conclusions moving forward.

CHAPTER NINE

RELATIONSHIPS

| THE MAJOR RELATIONS |

It is time to launch from the ground up with the most fuel-intensive part of our journey, our relationships. There are three major relationships in life:

1) How we are with ourselves: this comes down to how we feel about our survival and sexual nature, childhood traumas, sense of self-worth, insecurities, and mental movies.

2) How we are with others: how we feel about our romantic lives, family lives, and social lives.

3) How we are within society: how we feel about our roles and purpose in society, work, and overall ability to contribute and make a difference.

| PARENTAL |

We want to start with what came first. While you may think it was your relationship with yourself, your relationship with your parents existed before that. This is why we will explore our parental relationships first.

If we are serious about turning a light on and exposing the snakes in our life, we need to start with our relationships. Specifically, the ones we have with our parents. It is these beginning relationships that we want to explore because they set the foundation for how we interact with other people later in life. Until these issues are solved, all other relationships tend to suffer. It is like trying to fix your car without having any fuel in the tank. It does not matter how much time you spend working on your car, it is not able to be fully functional without fuel to start it.

The way you know if your relationship is solved is if the experience of it is whole, in that you do not need anything from them. You do not need them to change, approve of you, say this or that, or apologize. It is when you can relate to them without the sense that something is missing or tense. Experiencing them as they are, without need. This is a very rare experience for the majority of people and is why this section is dedicated to exploring it.

Previously, we explored the effect that our upbringing had on who we are and how we exist in the world. We explained that it was in your childhood where you learned a lot of the rules you live out today. What tends to happen with most people is we often become like one of our parents - usually, the one that we as a child thought had life figured out or who we perceived was in control. Due to this, our young minds started to emulate them and their way of being. This caused us to compulsively attempt to get the attention, approval, and care we wanted from them because to us, it felt like safety and survival. But if they were not in your life, you likely became the epitome of who you wanted them to be for you.

When these attempts did not work out, in that we never felt whole from our efforts to be like them, we ended up rejecting them and our similarities to them. This most likely caused a lot of tension and constant fighting growing up. There was a sense of power struggle or a disagreement in values in these arguments. Our desire to win the fights, prove them wrong, or cut them out of our lives comes from us trying to still get what we emotionally needed. Only this time by disempowering them or discrediting their worth so that their love and approval no longer held value. All of that is just us trying to be them but better. You accomplish this by either trying to convince them to be more like you or by you trying to fix their faults in yourself.

As the majority of us are unaware of these tendencies in ourselves, we never bother to question how they are working for us. Never examining how the mental movie of us proving them wrong or how we're better than them plays out. The truth is that this movie has already played out because it was never real to begin with. There is no possibility of a movie like that working out to make you right and them wrong. So, you are already aware that this strategy of living cannot make you "whole" or meet your needs.

Additionally, a lot of people believe their relationship with their parents is broken. This is nothing more than another movie in which a broken relationship gets fixed later or proves us right. As we have learned, this movie never gets to the good part. More often than not it even continues to play long after that parent has passed on. So, it is up to us to take on the responsibility of how these movies influence us. Allowing ourselves the realization that they have nothing to do with actually experiencing what we are after.

So, it is through observation of our relationship with them that we can see the reality of how we spend our experience in relation to them. We are not proving them wrong by cutting them out; we are only spending our life without parents. We are not teaching them a lesson on how they should have raised us; we are only wasting effort in trying to create an appearance of superiority. We are just experiencing them with a context that makes having our needs met impossible. That is it.

I'm not suggesting that you bring them back into your life, spend more time with them, or agree with them. This is just an invitation to explore how it would be if you let go of the movie of your parents being a certain way. It would play differently if instead, you realized there was no movie, to begin with. Only you relating to them from a context of survival that needs to prove them wrong. Again, this does not mean you need to agree with them, forgive them, ignore them, or engage with them. It only means that you allow yourself to observe how this movie influences your life, trying on for size the realization that you are already whole, to begin with. Realize that you do not need them to change or give you anything. Instead, becoming aware that their own limitations and flaws are just how they have learned to relate to their parents. This allows you to accept them as they are and give yourself the freedom to be whole and without need.

Regardless of the complications or tensions you do or do not have with your living or dead parents, it is worth exploring how much of your attention and effort is spent on the movie of proving your parents wrong or doing life better than they did so you are not them. This is not about forgiving them, but rather seeing how your need to be apologized to keeps you unhappy.

If this is not clear to you and you are sitting here thinking that your relationship with them is fine, I encourage you to honestly explore the following questions:

- What makes a perfect parent?
- How should a parent be with their child?
- How many of those answers come from what you feel you never received?
- Do you withhold your wellness from them so that they can continue to worry about you or to prove a point on how they messed up raising you?

- Do you feel a compulsion to exaggerate your accomplishments and brag about your life to get their approval or acceptance?

- Do you hold onto resentment for how they did not support you or believe in you when you needed them to?

- Is there a part of you that is not ok with how they are?

Again, these questions are not asked as a way to solve or change anything about your dynamic. Their purpose is to aid you in pointing out the movies that are playing, so you can determine whether they are productive to watch or not.

Another perspective we can take on how we relate to our parents is by understanding values. This is because the culture we grow up in influences what we come to value as important in life. At one point in our history, just making a living and keeping a roof over our heads was important. So, the values that came from that time were along the lines of just having work to do and making the most of tough times. Fast forward a few decades and you would see that being respected and accepted within your church or community was important. Now, the values would have been around keeping up with the neighbors and working for a reputable or prestigious company. Conflict happens when values clash. So compare those older values with modern values of purpose or passion in work. Older generations cannot accept those values as something to base your life on because it does not make sense based on the struggles they went through in achieving theirs.

We need to look at these differences not from a place of who is right and wrong but from an observation of our need to be right. Understanding that you are not supposed to change them because your parents existed before you. They lived in a different time of the world with a different culture which had different challenges that required different values. The fact that they do not share your values does not mean they do not approve of you. It does not mean they need to update their values, even if they are, in your judgment, ignorant, or uninformed. The differences in their upbringing and their values are equally as valid to their experience as your values are to your experience. In order for your values and way of life to exist, they had to be built from theirs. Like a strong foundation, it laid the opportunities and limitations that your values and lifestyles can then show up and engage with. This means without them holding the values, standards, and way of life they have, your way of life cannot exist. Additionally, would you want them to have to change their values at this point in their life? Would you want them to have to start from scratch in trying to make sense of the world as it is, denouncing all of their past as invalid? Really examine the extremeness of your need to feel right in life and how we tend to forget the consequences our tendencies cause in the lives of other people.

Values and differences aside, both parents and children want the same thing: to love and express that love. The hang-ups we have come from an inability to communicate what we feel because we get caught up in mental movies of how we have to be right. Just as we have them about our parents, they have them about their parents. Each generation passes down the limitations of how they learned to relate to their parents. When we observe these movies and the limitations they put on how we connect to our parents, we break the painful patterns in our families. If not for our parents to experience, then it can be for our own children to learn from moving forward.

All it takes is the responsibility to observe how we make ourselves limited in the experience of our parents. Then understanding that we do not need anything from them because our actual context is wholeness, and they can exist as they are without it meaning anything about us.

If you are truly committed to this process, it can be a valuable experience to do the following:

- Write a letter to them or call them and share how you have limited your relationship with them.
- In it, take responsibility for the movies you allowed yourself to believe.
- Communicate your appreciation for how they have shaped the positive parts of yourself.
- Finish your letter or conversation by committing to approach that relationship with the love you have for them moving forward.

Again, this is more for you than it is for them. So even if you write them a letter that you never send, the inner work is more important than trying to change the relationship. But if you do decide to send this, keep in mind that this can be very tough to both send and receive because this level of authenticity and communication is not common for people. Keep in mind that their reaction to this is not related to you, but about the limitations they hold with their own parents. Just know that all human beings want to love and be loved. It is only our inability to receive it that gets in our way. Thus, respect where they are, without needing to change them.

| PERSONAL |

OUR SEXUAL NATURE

Solving the internal relationship we have with ourselves ultimately comes down to how we relate to our sexual nature. This is because a large portion of our insecurities are formed from how we psychologically interpret our biological drive for sex. It is these insecurities that then heavily craft the identities and lives we live through. So, if we are serious about truly solving our internal relationship, we need to start with our sexual nature.

Every human being has had the experience of sexualizing another person with their thoughts. Maybe there is a recently hired person at your work or someone at your gym. Perhaps it was a quick thought about someone who got into the elevator you were in. This caused your mind to create images of the elevator getting stuck and the situation turning flirtatious. It could be with a barista or bartender you frequently see or a desire to pursue or be pursued by an acquaintance or stranger. These thoughts ignore responsibility and consequence. It could be ethical, unethical, moral, immoral, impulsive, or built up. It could be a new experience with your partner or infidelity. Regardless:

If you are mentally capable of deciding if someone is attractive or not, your thoughts are sexual in nature.

These thoughts can show up in many ways. It could be from an idea we get fixated on or one that is just fleeting. They might be repetitive or random thoughts, but they always show up without effort because of our minds. It is what allows us to judge the sexual value of a person and create narratives for sexual tension to occur. It is also what constructs visions and plays out the dynamics of a romance or passion that could unfold. While there are commonly shared ones, there are as many unique ones as there are people. This is because they come from the unlimited creativity of our imagination. Seeing as we all have imaginations, we can also conclude the following:

We are sex-craved perverts at our core.

The advertising industry knows it, religions know it, and we all intrinsically know it. It is why sex sells and why culture and religion obsess about it. Yet regardless of the many efforts to suppress, control, or stop these thoughts, they still emerge like perfectly timed clockwork in our minds. Due to our need to be considered socially appropriate, religiously moral, or fit our assumptions of what is typical, we judge these thoughts. We assume they mean something about us because they show up. As a result of our fantasies, we feel psychologically flawed, morally corrupt, or inherently ashamed.

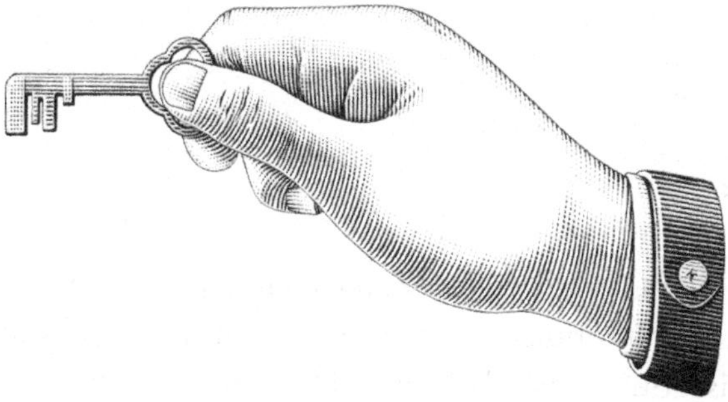

While you might have never given much thought to how or why these thoughts show up before, you most certainly experience emotions and behavior around managing them. This style of management often reflects one of two strategies for how we manage painful experiences in our life. From a young age, our minds learn to manage traumatic or painful memories by either expressing them in life or repressing them.

Take the unfortunate example of someone who has experienced sexual abuse. They tend to lean towards one of these strategies.

Repressing:

- They might try to hide the memory as a strategy to avoid it in the future, making anything sexual a forbidden topic they push away. This causes them to sensitize the meanings of their traumatic experience. This can cause them to refuse to talk about the experience or close themselves off to intimacy with new partners, essentially not 'going there' mentally. When a person chooses this strategy, they shut out and avoid anything that can be related to or trigger that experience. This way, they never have to face the pain they feel when their memory replays the movie in their mind.

Expressing:

- They might try to desensitize the memory as a strategy to weaken its emotional potency, such as engaging in hyper-promiscuous or risky behavior. They might crudely advertise themselves as a sexual object to attract more sexual activity to reduce the meaning of sex. When a person chooses this strategy, they actively pursue sex and perceive it as no big deal. This is because the more they engage in sex, the less it means. This makes all sexual behavior meaningless, including their traumatic experience. With this, the pain around that memory gets desensitized as it becomes just another meaningless act of sex.

While this is an extreme example, the act of choosing a strategy for managing our sexual thoughts remains the same. This starts when you are first exposed to sexuality, like:

- Seeing something explicit by accident as a child
- Feeling embarrassment when a parent corrects you for doing something inappropriate as a kid
- Recalling an experience of exploring your physical sensations as a kid, only to later realize it was sexual and feel shame for it
- Experiencing someone sexualize you

Regardless of how it started, these strategies then shape how we approach sexuality as an adult. Not just in how we manage our sex drive publicly but also how we judge others. Typically speaking, individuals who lean towards expression tend to place a lower importance on sex. Often judging other people as uptight, prudish, too formal, or old-fashioned. Alternatively, individuals who use a repression strategy tend to judge others who don't as damaged, immoral, promiscuous, or dirty.

These judgments are then used to base our experience of sex on. For example, if you negatively perceive others as promiscuous, you then experience your sense of worth as higher by refraining from sex. While this can create more self-respect as you deny yourself being casually used by people. It can also simultaneously create more anxiety and fear around having sex or performing well. This is similar to our concept of being overwhelmed from part two. But if you negatively judge others as prudish, you will be less inhibited sexually, thinking less about your ability because of your openness towards it. The downside of this is that sex can feel empty, cold, or mechanical, which can feel underwhelming or make a person feel hopeless in their romantic expectations.

Again, these judgments might be extreme, but your dependence on either strategy lives more on a spectrum. It is us that places sensitivity, or lack of it, on either side.

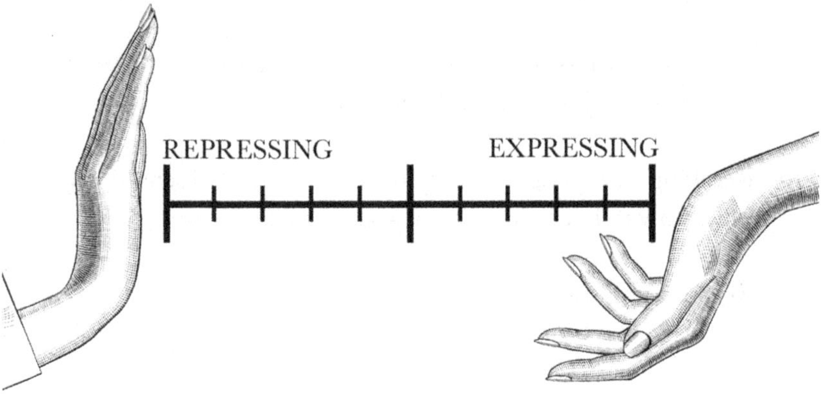

It is your place on this spectrum that will more often than not determine how you handle your sexual thoughts and fantasies. Some people hide their sexual thoughts from others, while others openly discuss them. Your place on this spectrum of sensitivity is also tied to your ability to experience romantic intensity and jealousy. If you have a tendency to repress, you will place more thought and meaning on sex. This creates more intense mental movies, allowing people to feel deep passion, attachment, and romance for someone. But this usually comes at the cost of also experiencing more jealousy, paranoia about infidelity, and a need for control. On the expression side of things, sex and relationships hold less importance which causes relationships to be more casual and meaningless. So, things like jealousy, obsessive thoughts, and a desire to control your partner no longer consume your mind.

Sticking to the premise of this book, we want to observe these tendencies as they are without meaning. We want to see neither strategy as better nor worse, only as a function of our mind. Once understood, this can be used as a tool to enhance our actual experience of life. If you can detach yourself from any judgment you feel towards other people, you can see them for where they are on a spectrum of sensitivity. No longer viewing them with the negative judgment you once had. Instead, you'll see the judgment that showed up as just a projection of your own need to manage your sexual thoughts. This means no longer judging others for being too prudish or promiscuous. Rather, seeing that judgment as our mind's way of justifying our own strategy.

When you are able to observe this type of judgmental thought happening, you stop your emotional attachment to being right. You start to see everyone around you as just doing the best they can. This enables you to connect with people on a deeper level. Additionally, you allow yourself the freedom from your own strategy, seeing your tendencies as just a reaction to a spectrum of sensitivity. With this, you can start to balance yourself on the spectrum. Willfully forcing the uncomfortable alternative strategy from a place of awareness so that you can improve your experience. This will remove the power of obsessive or anxious thoughts by expressing them through communication. Additionally, improving your sense of worth or passion by repressing and rejecting impulsive behavior.

All in all, our sexual thoughts just exist as a reaction of our minds. They are neither right, wrong, evil, normal, or any other meaning you could place on them. Just as our survival context paints meaning to things, our biological wiring for sex does the same. Only this time, our thoughts appear within a sexual context. This is how the mind naturally produces the many fantasies and compulsive sexual thoughts we have. The only issue with this is that:

Most people judge their biological desires as psychological issues.

But in reality, our sexual thoughts are nothing more than our mind's need to assign meaning to our physical impulses. Our biology is wired for sex, which means that we are naturally going to be drawn toward opportunities where that can happen. Like a heat-seeking missile focused on its target, our brain automatically looks for potential sexual partners. This wiring only cares about getting from A to B, with A being not having sex and B having sex. With this impulse, our mind's imagination fills the gap with how that could happen. Really think about this: while there are endless variations of different sexual thoughts and fantasies, they all share a common theme:

A fantasy is almost always the story or imagined circumstances which lead to a sexual encounter.

It is the story of how to get into or be in a sexual situation. It is just our mind's imagination playing with possibilities for the obtainment of sex. Fantasizing is nothing more than the way our mind presents options for obtaining and achieving our biological desires. If you can then observe this context in action and not demonize it or fear it motivating your actions, you can see it for what it is:

Just a biological drive interacting with a psychological imagination.

This awareness does not justify action or promote caution. Instead, it is just an opportunity to see yourself as you are without judgment. Simply by observing your sexual thoughts as just a function of your mind interacting with the body. That is it. So, trying to fight your imagination as though it is some sort of issue is like trying to charm a vulture off a carcass - a total waste of time.

JUDGING THE WORLD AROUND US

Our sexual context even produces thoughts to judge and assess social trends and the people who engage in them. While you might think you are accurate in how you judge what is popular or not, those thoughts are rarely based on anything other than your sexual context. You can see an example of this when you look at how you feel about things that are subjective in taste. Take for example:

- What type of fashion or style do you find ridiculous?
- What type of music or movies do you find irritating?
- Is there a type of terminology or slang that you consider unintelligent?
- How do you feel about a trend of behavior you see in younger people?
- What popular opinions do not make sense to you yet people believe them?
- Is there a social norm or attitude that logically does not make sense?

As you judge these things against your preferences, you will notice your way of being seems like the better option. This is because we often judge our experience of what is normal against other ways of being. We validate our preferences as the norm and the best way to live, and see alternatives as inauthentic, uncool, or less accurate. But in actuality, that judgment is just coming from our primal wiring. You can tell this by imagining those same things you once judged in a different light.

- Start by thinking of something that is considered trendy that you do not like.
- Entertain the idea of adopting that trend into your life and way of being.
- See it making you more fashionable, attractive, or valuable as you adopt it. Leading you to either get more sex, money, or popularity.

As you see yourself adopting that trend in your life, you might also feel yourself abandoning your judgment of that thing. This is because we are wired to take the path that best leads us to sex or survival. It can turn our judgment of "that is so ridiculous" into a justification of "I'm just keeping up with the times". Our mind creates rationalizations for that once judged trend the moment the primal reward becomes a possibility.

This is why we do not have a good sense of the overall marketplace of what is popular, only what we perceive to be. From this awareness of how our judgments are biased, we can start to release our need to understand and dismiss different ways of being. Doing this allows us the opportunity to be entertained by changes in culture, instead of feeling challenged by them. Now, this does not mean we need to involve ourselves in every new trend. Rather have the awareness to not judge it so confidently.

While this happens casually with subjective topics like fashion and taste, it also occurs in our beliefs and opinions of heavier topics like sex, politics, and religion. Most people tend to get opinionated on these topics as a way to justify and make sense of their own struggles. You can see this clearly when you look at how much their strongly held opinions rationalize their lack of sex, money, or popularity. We tend to become most opinionated and attached to our beliefs about the world when we do not feel successful. Alternatively, we have a tendency to be more relaxed and open-minded when we feel successful in our biological need for sex and survival. The point again is not to just chase after success as though it can bring happiness. Instead, it is to turn a light on the issue of what makes us unhappy. As our circumstances consistently change in life, so will the intensity of our opinions. This means:

The only real way to have contentment with our need to make others wrong is by recognizing our inability to be right.

NEGATIVE BELIEFS

As you read this book, you create a memory of the experience of reading it. It is a visual, audible, or kinesthetic sort of scene in which you mentally experience yourself flipping the pages and holding this book in your hands. You can remember all of the different points and insights and how they emotionally impacted you. When you are finished with this book, you will still be able to remember reading it because the experience of holding this book and reading these words was, in fact, a very tangible and real experience. So, imagine if someone came to you and told you that you did not read this book. You would not be able to logically agree with them. Based on your personal experience and memory, you would know that you held this book in your hands and read it at one point in time. This fact is not something you can believe did not happen. No matter how much effort they put into convincing you that you never read it, you would still know as a fact that you did read it.

This example is a lot like how we experience our beliefs about who we are, more particularly the ones related to our self-worth and insecurities. Regardless of what people tell us, the achievements we make, or the mantras we tell ourselves, our beliefs about ourselves are a very real experiences for us. Like the book example, we often emotionally feel what we factually know. So regardless of how much positive thinking we do or praise we get, a negative belief we have about ourselves still seems very real and factual to us. The reason for this is because our beliefs about what is real come from our experience in life. Just like knowing for a fact that you read this book, our beliefs about who we are come from past experiences we know we had.

This is also why most of us can remember a time in which our insecure belief started. Maybe it was a moment in school when the other kids treated you poorly or a teacher criticized you. Perhaps it was an experience with a parent or relative when they yelled at you or did not make time for you. Maybe you tried something and failed, or you missed an opportunity because you felt scared in the moment. Regardless, the negative beliefs we hold about ourselves start from one or multiple experiences we can point to.

The challenge with beliefs is that they feel as real as the memories they came from. Meaning that you either believe it or you do not. There is no partial belief when it comes to what we emotionally feel. You can see this when you recite a belief about yourself that is not true, like, "I am a giraffe." When you read and say that to yourself, it emotionally feels like nothing because you know it is untrue. But that is not the case for many people when they read these common negative beliefs:

- "I am not worthy of love"
- "If I fail, I will not be loved"
- "I am not enough"
- "I am not important"
- "I am ugly"
- "I do not belong"

If you felt a slight fear, worry, or other emotional reaction that was not like the giraffe statement, this is because the belief is real to you on some level. Even if you have spent time working on this insecurity or issue, a belief is as real to us as the experience that started it. This is why most positive thinking strategies and cognitive reframes never fully solve it. Instead, they cause a person to constantly experience new situations that confirm it, which then only strengthens the belief further.

Instead of doing this, we can use observation and the insights from this book to deconstruct negative beliefs. Permanently eradicating them and completely removing the constant suffering they cause. This is not with some anti-intellectual tactic in which we pretend to convince ourselves of something that we do not actually believe. Instead, it can be done by taking the time to explore each negative belief in ourselves, one by one.

We have to realize that most of these beliefs started when we were very young. During that time, our minds were more egotistical and focused on our own feelings and meanings. Considering our younger age, we made the most logical decision at the time. Using our survival context, we assigned meaning to the circumstance and how it negatively related to us. Despite the fact that this might seem like a logical interpretation on which to base our belief, it is ultimately limited compared to our present abilities.

While it is easy to just read this next part and intellectually grasp it, allow yourself to emotionally commit to the process. Complete and ask these questions to yourself. Even though it is a simple process, it is one that we have to do ourselves if we want to truly experience freedom from our negative beliefs.

Complete these steps in your head or write your answers down.

- Start by pointing to a negative belief you have about yourself.
- Identify the earliest memory you have that made you believe this.
- Allow yourself to fully remember how you felt and the sensations of it.
- Imagine how other random people would have described the event if they were in the room and watched the experience unfold.
- Think about some possible alternative interpretations that they could make from watching you go through that (such as just watching people talking, just kids being kids, or just a parent who is busy or stressed).
- Do you think they would interpret that belief as something you should have? or is it possible that they do not have your interpretation?
- Is your interpretation objective or subjective then?
- Rather than point out the event itself, try to SEE the belief.
- Where can you *SEE* the belief?
- Notice that your mind returns to the event which is real, but is unable to actually locate the belief as a real thing.
- If a new event comes up as evidence for the belief, repeat the process until you realize that you are unable to see the belief, only the meaningless events.
- Keep questioning and attempting to point to the belief as a real thing until it starts to dismantle itself as separate from the events that once supported it.

This process requires commitment. But once you do this, it should feel a lot like a belief that no longer makes sense emotionally. Such as learning that Santa is not real or being given new information that debunks old information. Once a belief is dismantled, it rarely returns. This is because now what is real is the awareness you have of how meaning is separate from content. As well as how our mind paints meaning onto inherently meaningless experiences. When you realize this, you do not only see the irrationality of these negative beliefs, but you no longer feel them as valid because they cannot be. With this, the mind cannot unsee what it has seen and you would now have to lie to yourself to keep this belief alive.

The true realization of this is to become aware of all subjective beliefs, both good and bad. Realizing that both disempowering beliefs and naively empowering ones are not grounded in experience. While you may be tempted to hold onto ones you perceive as positive, your attachment to them can only ever limit your experience. This will lock you into a limited identity that never fully uses your full potential. You will notice this if you feel a compulsive feeling to defend and repeatedly prove this belief to yourself and others. Constantly attempting to demonstrate this belief as true, when in actuality it only limits our ability to learn and blinds us with wishful, subjective thinking. In essence, it keeps true experiences which are "whole in nature" trapped behind a movie that we are trying to feel validated by. So, it is time to leave the theatre of our mind and build our sense of worth from the "wholeness" that we are, despite thinking we are not.

| PASSIONATE |

OUR IDEALS

Think about your ideal romantic relationship. If you are in one then it's the changes you would like to see. If you are single then it is the relationship you are attempting to get. As you think about this scenario, allow yourself to see exactly what you would like as though a genie would be able to grant exactly what you wanted. Right now, answer the following questions honestly.

- What changes in your relationship would you need in order to be completely and totally satisfied?
- What would you like them to stop doing or do more of?
- How would you like to feel in your relationship and what type of emotions are you after?
- What labels in your relationship do you need to have in order to feel satisfied? (Taken? Exclusive? Casual? Married?)
- What circumstances do you feel you need to have to be happy? (Homeowner? Parents? Engaged?)
- What behaviors would you need to see from your partner to know they loved or respected you?
- What does not work within your relationship that irritates and upsets you?
- What's not fair about your current relationship?
- What could your partner do to be better for you?
- Do you want more intimacy, trust, loyalty, or communication?

After thinking about this list, you should have at least an idea of the gap between where you are with your relationships and where you wish you could be. While this gap could be big or small, what is certain is that the gap describes what we believe are the reasons behind our dissatisfaction with our relationships. It shows that very rarely do we truly feel content, complete, and genuinely satisfied with our relationships. This dissatisfaction seems to create a filter or block between truly connecting with our partner. We believe that if only these issues, irritations, wants, demands, or needs could change, we would be able to experience a more profound sense of connection and love. It is this gap that seems to cause us to:

- Not fully commit to the success of the relationship
- Refusing to be vulnerable or open up completely
- Reject love and affection over making a point or communicating our dissatisfaction
- Become resentful and emotionally distant
- Hold onto past problems or mistakes as justifications for punishment
- Be unwilling to forgive or accept someone for who they are as they are
- Obsessively desire new partners or continually question the relationship
- Remain on the lookout for better relationships or constantly compare yours to others
- Become closed off to experience because of an idea of standards or must-haves

While this gap of dissatisfaction might feel logical or valid, it is only another by-product of your survival context. So, while you might think you know exactly what you want, your desire for change is nothing more than another mental movie in which you later become satisfied. The issue with the movie of our relationships is that it seems more factual in that we believe we know what we want because of our ability to recall the past or imagine the future. We believe that because we can remember what we disliked or enjoyed about past relationships, we have a good sense of what we want in future ones. On top of this, we then have a very clear imagination that lets us perceive a desired future of how we think our ideals will feel once we get them. But, both previous experience and perceived future experience come from our imagination's ability to create a mental movie that is not an experience itself. These gaps and the dissatisfaction of our relationships is the result of our inability to reference actual experience. This is because we only ever reference the movies we think represent the experience.

VIEWING ROMANCE

This issue can be easily understood when we look at a romantic film you might watch in the theatre. When you watch the romance, you see the two characters go through a summary of events that led them to falling in love. These events are filmed with big panoramic scenes, close-ups of the actors, and beautiful cinematography. Then before it is shown to you, an editor collects the best shots and adds background music that provokes emotional highs and lows to match the story. All of this is then compiled into a highlight reel that paints a romantic narrative over the events that unfolded for these characters. We might see them on their first date with a scene of them both nervously getting ready, then cutting to the scene where they meet at the restaurant. Next, it cuts to a scene of them giving their orders to the waiter. This is followed by a montage of the night unfolding in laughter and flirtation until the end of the date when they kiss goodbye. While this was an entire night for the characters, it was viewed in under a few minutes for us. Part of masterful storytelling is being able to tell an entire life story in under a few hours. This is done by highlighting the key moments and summarizing the events of the characters. But if we were to imagine how the characters actually felt going through those experiences, it would be very different from how we experienced it as a viewer. We do not experience the moment-by-moment dullness of their actual first-person experience of life in between cuts. For example, when they spent 30 minutes in traffic to get to the restaurant thinking random thoughts in their heads. As well as how they silently read the menu so they could figure out what they wanted to eat without cinematography and background music painting the scene. The actual second-by-second experience of being on that date as a character is very different from our experience as a viewer watching a romance unfold. They have no context to their life and how it fits into the story of a romance, only experiencing life as it happens.

While this seems obvious, this distinction is important. It identifies the difference between the actual experience of being on that date versus the experience of watching an emotional film as a viewer. It is us viewing our mental movies as how we should feel versus the actual emotions that you would experience having those circumstances come true. This matters because the imagined emotions of romance that many people wish they had tends to be what they base their life on. These experiences are not even achievable for the characters, let alone for us. So like the director and editor of the film, we go through a similar process of editing our memories of the past and imaginations of the future. We create and watch mental movies that play out like a highlight reel of how we imagine that different situation or circumstance as being. All of which are nothing like how those circumstances are experienced in the moment.

The real issue is that our mind's imagination buys into these mental movies as valid dissatisfactions when they are really just imagined. This means that even if we could get our partner to stop being late or commit more, our satisfaction won't come from these external changes. This is because as we picture our partner meeting our imagined ideals our emotions are based on that imagery, not on the actual experience. Those emotions from our mental movies are never possible for us to have while we live in our first-person experience. It is like expecting us to have our emotions as viewers be the same as the emotions of the character on the date. This is like us becoming obsessed with trying to experience living the concept of "happily ever after". So similarly our satisfaction is impossible regardless of attaining everything we think we wanted. This really comes down to:

You have no idea what you want in the future; you only have imaginations.

This is because most of us base our ideals on things we think we want which have nothing to do with how those circumstances are actually experienced. So while you might feel certain that you need to get married, have kids, be with someone who never snores, or whatever other dissatisfactions you feel you need to solve; none of that has anything to do with your ability to be satisfied in your relationships. This is because satisfaction is a context. It's like a paint bucket that paints the content of your life with the awareness that you are whole and need nothing to change. This causes you to experience you, your partner, and life as they are with a commitment to keeping focused on how your current experience relates to your satisfaction. Instead of defaulting to our mind's survival context of dissatisfaction.

The real reason you are dissatisfied in your relationships is because you are unsatisfiable.

SATISFIED

When you show up in your relationship with a survival context of dissatisfaction, you stay there because you believe that your demands, wants, and standards are valid. You believe you can achieve them and that they can give you the satisfaction you want. The issue is that they have nothing to do with satisfaction because that is a context and awareness that you internally bring to the relationship.

Answer the following question honestly once more:

What do you believe you need in order to be satisfied?

Now imagine you got the mental movie you wanted with every demand or issue solved on your list. Be it marriage, kids, a partner who does not complain, or whatever it is for you.

- Is it a possibility that you could experience a totally passionate and fulfilling relationship in which those things are not in your life?
- Is it a possibility that you could have those things yet be totally dead inside?
- Could you have those things and be lacking passion or the love you thought it would bring?

Despite all of these changes, it is still a possibility that you could end up dissatisfied. In fact, more often than not people do get what they think they want. Only to find themselves feeling that same experience of dissatisfaction that ignited those wants. This is the experience of either wishing for more pleasure or less pain in the future. It is very possible that the things you think you want do not end up making you satisfied. Alternatively, it is also very possible that other experiences that you never imagined on your list end up being very satisfying. This is because:

Satisfaction does not come *from* experiences, but rather by being *open to* experience as it is.

It is through our commitment to accept circumstances, issues, and people as they are that we find satisfaction. We can enter relationships from a place of already being satisfied, solved, and complete. This is being aware of our wholeness and experiencing life without need. It is seeing our relationships as opportunities to connect and relate instead of challenges and issues to change. It is choosing to love people fully as they are without needing them to be lovable. It starts with our observation of how our mind creates dissatisfaction. It is being aware that our survival context makes us dissatisfied and that solving those issues cannot lead to the satisfaction we seek. So, instead of buying into our dissatisfaction as valid and getting consumed in solving it, we instead observe our minds creating this dissatisfaction from a distance.

Understand that our satisfaction comes from accepting that our mind does this as a survival function. However, it does not have to be taken as valid.

This is not about wishful thinking and pretending bad things do not happen in life. Instead, we recognize that our control in life comes from our commitment to accept life as it comes and not get caught up in complaining about what is not. This is where you concern yourself with the opportunity to relate instead of complain. Allowing yourself to experience emotions of love and deep connection in your relationship as it is. Where you stop waiting for it to be an ideal that it never could be because you understand your mind is incapable of accurately predicting the future.

This way of approaching relationships has nothing to do with trying to see the positives in a person or pretending you do not have problems. Instead, it is about understanding that your control is in your reaction to the reaction. So, if something like jealousy shows up as a reaction, you remain open to it as an experience without needing to assign meaning to it. It is just part of what showed up; it does not mean it should not be there or needs to change; it just is. Experience it as an opportunity to relate and communicate what you feel from a place of sharing, instead of placing pressure on another person to fix it. It is about taking responsibility for your experience. You do this by communicating without making them feel wrong about something. Allow yourself the opportunity for you to authentically relate to someone without needing them to change. It's about giving yourself the possibility to relate in a way that goes beyond pointing out your dissatisfaction.

Here is a practical example of this. Imagine your partner has a very annoying trait where they chew with their mouth open. Most people's automatic reaction is to relate to them in the form of a complaint or passive aggressive comment aimed at getting them to stop. As you learn to show up with satisfaction as a context, you start by seeing your irritation as part of how your brain keeps you dissatisfied. You are aware that you will still feel dissatisfied even if your imagined movie of them not chewing out loud actually gets experienced. You know that your viewing of their trait comes from a context of dissatisfaction which has nothing to do with them and everything to do with you. In that, your communication changes to one in which you take responsibility for your experience by saying, "I do not know why but I feel irritable and little things are bothering me. Even small things that shouldn't be a problem, seem to be. Do you ever feel that way or have any insights on that?". With this type of communication, you have opened up a possibility for you to authentically relate to them, instead of just complaining. As a result, a productive or a funny conversation could occur which would lead to more satisfaction than any attempt at reducing the dissatisfaction would.

When you show up to your relationship with a commitment to satisfaction, you become satisfiable. In that, you experience an openness to your partner as they are. You experience your time with them as an opportunity to love and relate to one another instead of wasting it with bickering, complaining, or resentment over some mental movie of what it is not.

This is a realization that your relationship problems, wants, issues, and dissatisfaction are how you choose to relate.

All of this has nothing to do with actually experiencing contentment or happiness in that moment.

It is in your moments of relating to your partner as they are that you disconnect from your dissatisfaction.

Allow yourself to fully experience something for what it could be and how it might unfold instead of limiting that moment with your judgment because of what it is not. This is positive because it is in your moments of fully experiencing a situation with openness that we can end up surprised, inspired, and profoundly impacted. This is what we are ultimately after when we get down to why we even buy into our dissatisfaction to begin with. One of the best examples of our desire to relate, rather than fix dissatisfaction, can be found in the intimacy we have with our partner.

No one in the heat of relating with passionate intimacy has ever been upset about who did the dishes last.

This is because what we are really after is relating, not just sexually but in all variations. When we approach interactions with a context of satisfaction, we see them as opportunities to relate physically, emotionally, intellectually, spiritually, or any other variation of expression. As a person learns to approach relationships this way, their demeanor expresses one of non-judgment and openness. This allows space for people to relate as they are and not just as another dissatisfied person. This ironically attracts the very things that other people use as their wants and must-haves. The reason for this is that marriage, kids, or whatever else you want are better experienced as a reaction to two people who have built up the habit of relating for sake of satisfaction. Then from a context of satisfaction, their experience of relating organically expands and develops into marriage or kids. It does this as a complement to their dynamic instead of two separate individuals both trying to get out of their inherent dissatisfaction.

Regardless of whether you are dating or single, make a commitment to experience and relate to people from a context of satisfaction. Focus your attention on simply remaining open to the possibilities of relating with them. Observe experience itself without your mind's need to get to an outcome or change something. Just exist with that person as you and they are. If it is enjoyable while interacting and relating with them, do more. If not, do less. The fact is, that is all there ever will be. Ironically if you can do this, the common result is people's desire to build a life with you. Which marriage, kids, or the courtesy of not chewing out loud tends to occur. Only this time, it will be because you genuinely approach experience without the need for them to be a certain way. You understand that those things are better experienced as a possibility of relating and not as achievements to get.

This openness to experience and approach to life with a context of satisfaction could mean you release your hesitation towards commitment or the need to be free. This is because you have no idea what you want and neither does anyone else. Imagining how you will feel in the future has nothing to do with actually experiencing the experience. This can look like a person thinking they do not want kids, yet later finding themselves in an enjoyable relationship with a person and wanting to expand that relating into parenthood. This is all because their experience of relating has been so enjoyable that they naturally desire to expand together. But sadly and more often than not, this can also mean that people who thought they wanted a family life and marriage find themselves not enjoying life. Wishing they had not forced this outcome as the actual experience itself has nothing to do with the mental movie they previously imagined. This is why:

When you stop trying to get your perfect relationship, you can start enjoying one.

RELATING

The biggest realization of this comes down to understanding the limiting way we often show up for our partners. Most people think they *have* a relationship in that it is something they can point to and physically identify. But:

You cannot *have* a relationship, you can only *experience* one.

This means it is only when you relate to someone that you experience a relationship. Outside of that, you have a transaction. What most people believe is their relationship is nothing more than a mental movie about how they met, what they do, and stories of their past - none of which has anything to do with relating. This is not to discredit that movie or the emotions replaying it can create. It is only to distinguish the movies against what is actually experienced in the current moment versus what is just mentally thought. We want to do this because most people think their relationship instead of experiencing it. This means they spend more time trying to protect and keep their relationship as though it is a tangible thing they have instead of focusing on relating to their partner so that a relationship can be experienced.

Because this distinction is not clear for most people, they interpret experiencing a relationship as having something. This is what leads people to obsessing over relationship labels, trying to figure out where it is going or attempting to decipher how serious or casual it is. All of this is just our biological survival wiring trying to keep what gives us pleasure. All while trying to avoid the pain of losing it and figuring out ways to maximize this effect while minimizing the effort required to do so.

Most people relate by trying to not get hurt rather than trying to add more pleasure.

This creates a habit of trying to maintain their idea of a relationship by means of a transaction in which they attempt to trade gestures, statements, and effort. This is a way to keep a person from leaving the relationship. This looks a lot like the difference of:

Saying "I love you" as a form of relating and articulating an experience of love being felt

vs

Saying "I love you" as a statement you expect to hear in return so you feel like your transaction of not hurting each other is safe

---

Giving a gift because you felt inspired to surprise and please them

vs

Giving a gift because it was expected for an occasion or as a way of apologizing so they do not exit the transaction

---

Wanting to work through an issue they have as a way to refocus their mind on what is important because you are committed to being their partner in self-actualization

vs

Wanting to work through an issue because you are afraid they will leave you or the relationship will end if you do not

This is why most relationships are unsuccessful, even if the people remain together in a transaction.

Relationships based on ways to avoid pain often lack possibilities for pleasure.

In order to protect ourselves from pain, we tend to build relationships that limit pleasure to just the absence of pain. Reducing the experience of a relationship to one that spends our energy trying not to get hurt instead of how to build more passion.

This is why we get hung up and obsessed about what has to happen or how people have to act before we allow ourselves to be satisfied. Like believing we will let go of past resentments once a person apologizes, or that we will put effort into the relationship when they do. All of these occur because we start with a flawed premise. This states if we can get some satisfaction out of our partner and they can get some satisfaction out of us, that constitutes a good relationship. But while this might seem logical, it is almost always a recipe for failure. This is because when we keep satisfaction as something external from us, we can only ever take from our relationships in order to be happy.

A relationship can only be a success if it is a place in which people go to give, not get.

Until then, it is just a transaction that is locked in rules and metrics around what is expected and how to not get hurt. This is the real reason most people are dissatisfied in their relationships. This is because they get caught up in the dissatisfaction of stories about what is not fair or how they deserve better. They believe in a movie where their partner apologies, changes, or gives them satisfaction as though that was part of the deal. When in reality, they are only ever holding satisfaction in the distance because their context of dissatisfaction makes them believe satisfaction is not their responsibility.

CHAPTER TEN
WORK

| WORKING FOR OTHERS |

Just as we cannot experience our ideal relationship using the standards of our imagined mental movies, the same goes for our ideal job. As our imagination thinks of the future, it paints an image of what our ideal career will feel like. But once we actually get what we think we want, it tends to not resemble what we previously expected, just like in the example of the young woman who got her ideal job at the law firm. The experience of work for most people is one of either overwhelm or underwhelm but rarely contentment or happiness. It is the experience of waiting for the promotion, waiting for the job offer, waiting for the raise, or waiting for the opportunity. None of these actually makes any lasting difference to the quality of our life from a moment-to-moment basis once we acquire it.

This is not to say that more financial security or improved living conditions cannot bring enjoyment. However, more often than not our need for them creates a never-ending chase instead of satisfaction, regardless of what we do for work. So, when we look at these needs for a better career or more meaningful work, we have to understand where it is coming from. For most people, their desires come from an identity they hold which keeps them from facing their insecurities and internal snakes. This means your identity tends to set a standard for you to uphold in order for you to accomplish your avoidance of pain. This standard is the role or job you should have in order to be worthy of love or achieve the imagined approval of others. So, it is common to find our identities influencing what we think we need, such as:

- Achievers need to achieve in their work
- Teachers need to be seen as knowledgeable
- Helpless people need to avoid responsibility
- Helpers need to focus on others

It is in these identities that we create lives that might not reward us from an experience perspective. So, it often happens that:

- Achievers hate the experience of constantly needing achievement
- Teachers dislike having to always know everything
- Helpless people want an opportunity to take charge
- Helpers would rather focus on themselves

It is through our identities and how they are validated by others that we create the prison we spend our efforts trying to maintain. This happens because as we think of how to make ourselves happy, we often look towards how our identity could double down on what it has done so far. This forces our minds to create a mental movie of how we could further validate and crystalize how we have come to be. The main way it does this is with our work.

While you might think that your desire to start a business or get into a prestigious profession is something you have picked through extensive thought, more often than not it came from the movie of what you think that job will feel like. Then depending on which path glorifies or validates your identity more, that is how you determine which path you believe is right for you - similar to how advertisers sell alcohol. They typically show you imagery of fun parties, easy sex, and luxury. In this same way, we hold grandiose images of what we think we will be like and feel once we become a doctor, lawyer, or successful entrepreneur. It is an imagination of the respect and admiration people will have for us once we finally get that title or result. But in reality, this is just a mental movie that is stroking our ego.

While we can have our ego rewarded and praised by people in our lives for these accomplishments, the praise eventually wears off and the glory fades in comparison to the day-to-day reality of maintaining it. It might sound extreme to suggest that this is the case. However, if a person really looks into why they actually want their job, it would likely come down to some variation of the following statement.

Most people choose their profession based on how it validates their existence, instead of how the time experiencing it would be spent.

While this is not the case for everyone, it is the case for many who do not have satisfaction with their work. If you have uncertainty in your professional life or feel dissatisfaction towards the work, it is because you are unaware of the difference between the identity of that job and the actual experience of it.

Another way to prove that this is the case is to look at how you experience motivation when trying to learn or do something new. It is common for people to find that their motivation disappears as they tell people about what they are trying to accomplish before doing it. It is almost as though the motivation they had to learn a new skill disappeared once they told someone about their attempts at learning it. This is because most of our desires to improve come from trying to validate our identity or maintain it. Once we receive praise for our ambition from telling people, our motivation to actually complete it goes away. This is because what we were after wasn't the new skill or achievement but the validation that comes from praise. We interpret this as us keeping our insecurities and snakes away.

So, answer these questions honestly about your current job or ideal job.

Do you enjoy how your day and time are actually spent with your profession?

If no one knew you did this, would you still enjoy it?

Do the behaviors of your work feel fulfilling and meaningful?

If you had to redo your training or education to get this position, would you?

Do you believe you would let others down if you decided to pursue a humbler task?

Do you want the identity of the job or the experience of it?

The key here is not to make any judgments about ourselves or how we got here. Instead, it is to only question our motivation for maintaining it. We do this so that we can gain awareness of the part of ourselves that creates dissatisfaction. Emotionally understanding that:

The identity of a job can never fulfill you, only the actual experience of it can.

This comes down to how we actually spend our time doing that work. The second-by-second sensation of getting lost in it. Our moment-by-moment enjoyment of the work. It is only through our ability to lose ourselves, meaning the thoughts we think we are, that we find true contentment. When we learn to experience our work just for us, as a sensation and not as a validation, we can find true enjoyment in what we do.

Refocusing on the experience of your work can be difficult if it is not enjoyable for you. Take for example our young woman who became a lawyer. While the praise from her family and friends was nice and she has a prideful feeling as she gets to tell people she is a lawyer that only makes up a very small percentage of her second-by-second life. It would be five minutes here and there every month, totaling to at most twenty minutes of validation per month. The rest of her life is actually spent reading old case files and doing paperwork which she actually finds tedious and unenjoyable. This is how a lot of us approach our work in life. We do so as a means to maintain an identity which is a collection of behaviors and beliefs that try to hide insecurities and fears that do not even exist. Then, we use the few brief moments of avoiding the snake to justify the largest unenjoyable part of how we spend our time on this earth. So, while this might feel like some epic movie where you get to go to your high school reunion with confidence having proved your bullies wrong with all your success. Or perhaps you get to rub it in your parent's faces for their lack of support. It is really just us as fully grown adults, living our life in a dissatisfied way. That is it. Realistically, you'd be trying to prove a point that no one was actually arguing against you with anyway.

People are so hyper-concerned with their own lives that they forget they are actually in other people's. Really think about this: do you know of anyone currently trying to prove you wrong with their dissatisfaction? Probably not.

This is why it is essential for us to become aware of how much of our life and work is based around these movies and identities. We can then start to make a more conscious decision to enjoy our experience as though it is all we get. The way you experience your life at this moment, with the job you have and the life you are living, is simply what it is.

This right now is the great show of life. There is no rehearsal. You are on stage so make it your favorite performance.

| PROBLEMS, PROJECTORS & PURPOSE |

The goal is to be able to distinguish the difference between what part of our interpretation of work is experienced and what part is imagined. Once we can observe this, we can start to distance ourselves from the imagined movies that used to influence it. This is not about radically changing your career or quitting your job to go get a new one. Because this awareness is just the first part.

We get into these situations unconsciously and non-deliberately, which means even if you leave your job now, you will often find yourself in a similar situation in a matter of months. Take for example the classic story of someone quitting their job in the corporate world to pursue a creative inspiration. While they had a very stable 9-5 job with great benefits and pay, they decided to quit because they became aware of their dissatisfaction. Part of what motivated their decision was just another movie in which they get to now do what they love as a creative. Even though at the time they could justify the financial insecurity, longer hours, and a reduction in their lifestyle, they failed to realize that those justifications were made from a place that did not experience those. So a few years later, those once justified sacrifices were now contributing to a new dissatisfaction in which they wished for the best of both worlds. While they were correct to observe their dissatisfaction in this example, they only really traded one movie for another.

The second part, of this awareness is recognizing that this dissatisfaction is inherent in all outcomes until you learn to observe it. Changing your external circumstances without changing your internal condition will only contribute to your dissatisfaction. So while it might temporarily relieve your dissatisfaction, that relief was more likely due to your belief that you have progressed in your mental movie. But, in our moments of transition, we break our cognitive habits and are forced to go with the flow and momentum of the situation. This is because with a rapid change of stimulus, our brain shifts away from trying to place meaning and returns to just trying to watch and spot patterns. The result is that we are no longer overthinking and are finally able to get out of our own heads. With this, we overwhelmed the thinking mind with new sensations. In this period, we are forced to have a greater sense of openness to the world. Possibility because we are not familiar with the challenges of the new movie.

While this might seem good, it is not practical to maintain a theme of running away from any form of habit or dissatisfaction. Instead, we're better off to observe and understand why we have this tendency to return to dissatisfaction as a default. Being able to recognize this tendency in our thinking is the key to gaining awareness of it. When you can see how you continue this pattern, regardless of the circumstance, you can start to really point to it as an experience we put ourselves through. You can also observe the act our mind makes in forcing thoughts to come up, recognizing the difference between what is interpreted and what is experienced.

The experience *is* our mind producing thoughts.

By observing the thoughts of "I am unhappy at my job", and recognizing that those thoughts are not "you" giving that assessment. But instead, this is just the way the mind interacts with the observer. By understanding this you can then start to have some control over your experiences. This is really how we start to gain control of dissatisfaction. By remembering that:

It is not that *we have* thoughts about what is accurate and truthful, but instead that our thoughts *have us*.

This observation and awareness of our subjectivity is required before any sort of satisfaction can occur. We cannot change our experience of satisfaction from the level of thought that creates dissatisfaction. This is why trying to think your job is enjoyable when you have already perceived that it is not, cannot work at an emotional level. At most, you can only end up suppressing your thoughts and ignoring your emotional signals. Which is not what we are aiming to do.

Once we can distance ourselves from our mind's tendency to put thoughts in our head, seeing it as just a mechanism, we can recognize that our thoughts are not actually a productive thing to observe. Only until this happens, the observer can then either watch those thoughts up close, like sitting in a theater seat. Or from a distance, like being in the projector room watching the movie project onto the screen. From that place, we can actually have a choice:

Do nothing and allow our focus to naturally return us to our theatre seats to continue watching the movie

or

Willfully decide to experience a movie from the glass window of the projector room

When we willfully allow ourselves to watch a movie, the movie becomes a choice. It becomes an experience in which we can appreciate things from a different perspective. One that observes thoughts as entertainment for us to select from. Analogy aside, it is us fully accepting that our mind creates thoughts and that they are nothing but imagined meanings being painted overtop of our current job. If this is an inevitable part of being human, we might as well enjoy the show for what it is. When we approach our lives in this way, we experience satisfaction. However, it has to come from the willful acceptance of our mind placing context as something we have no control in. As a result, we need to know that we can return our attention to the projector room to observe the difference between our subjective thoughts and our objective circumstances. When this awareness is had, we can recontextualize our circumstance from a context of satisfaction. Seeing our current job as an opportunity to contribute and experiencing it as a place we can go to add and actualize our potential within. From this context of satisfaction, we can make a difference because we see it as a place that allows us to expand ourselves within. In that, we now look for new ways to solve the limitations of it, experiencing it like a challenge for us to rise to. Again, this is only possible if we first deconstruct how *we* make it dissatisfying. Once we understand our role in that process, we can then approach the same circumstance with a more productive meaning - one that is resourceful and looks for how this can fit into your life as a good thing. When you come from this willful place, you look for how you can contribute and make a difference, instead of the previous dissatisfying context. Which made you assume that your work's satisfaction and purpose was something externally created. When you truly grasp that it is you that makes a job meaningful or not, you will almost always choose to approach it with as a place you can contribute to.

When we do this, we also experience purpose in our work. This is because we approach our work with the awareness that our purpose is not something you find or get from some particular circumstance. In that, our purpose can be found from some situation over another.

Purpose is just a reaction we get to contribution.

So, as we approach our job like an opportunity to contribute, we simultaneously experience the purpose many people feel at a loss for.

CHAPTER ELEVEN
LIFE

| RECONTEXTUALIZING LIFE |

When we look back on the many topics of this book, we can start to get a clearer picture on how happiness, motivation, and purpose show up for us. They first start by an awareness and deconstruction of what causes unhappiness. Then, from that place of observation, a new context can be placed for our minds to create meaning from. It can be a context of wellness, abundance, contribution, or wholeness. This proactive context has us approach our experience in life differently than how we once did. Instead of being engulfed in the drama of ups and downs that once consumed our attention we use our mental facilities of memory and imagination to take a more empowered meaning. The result of this is a reaction of more happiness, motivation, and purpose that was previously hidden under the noise of our previous dissatisfaction. Satisfaction in life is had as a consequence of this.

This is not to suggest that life will no longer have ups and downs or that we are in some way not to experience negative emotion. All of which will still occur, as challenges and obstacles are a natural part of life. However, it is our responsibility to keep an awareness of what is objectively vs. subjectively interpreted in our lives. Meaning, it is up to us as observers to cultivate this ability so we can free ourselves from rules and fears that no longer serve us. Committing to an inquiry on our beliefs and mental movies by questioning the actual experience they provide, instead of what we think they will lead us to.

That is because this experience we are currently living is what we get from life, not the movie or interpretation.

Really commit to re-asking and re-examining the questions in this book. Because as you seriously consider the role you play in the limitations you feel towards your emotions, relationships, and work, you change the experience you have towards them.

When we stop closing ourselves off to what life is by thinking of what life is not, we open ourselves up to what life could be.

This is where our power is, through the ability to recontextualize life as an opportunity to engage with, so that our meanings show up as more empowering ones. As a result, we experience more motivation, purpose, and ultimately more contentment.

| FIVE STAGES OF AWARENESS |

As a person approaches life in this way, they go through different phases of awareness. While you might not start at the beginning, your place on this does not matter as this is more of a map to explore, than a race to finish. There are five stages of awareness that a person progresses through, with each stage representing a different level of observation occurring. The higher the stage, the more able they are to deconstruct how their thoughts show up, seeing them as less real. The lower they are, the closer and more engaged they are to their thoughts, experiencing their interpretations as more visceral and accurate. But, because of our biological proclivities, maintaining any given stage usually does not happen, as we jump from stage to stage during different periods of our life. While our commitment to maintaining a high level of awareness can greatly influence the stage we are at, the amount of effort required to maintain this commitment can be high. Taking into account our biology's survival drive to minimize effort while maximizing the result, our minds are influenced to hide and forget this commitment. The purpose of this is in an attempt to reduce the energy required in sustaining this awareness. This is why we can often have moments of very deep enlightenment and clarity but also return to moments of stupidity and ignorance.

The goal is to understand that while it is natural for us to be aware, that ability coexists with a stronger natural drive to reduce effort, which causes unawareness. That is why we need to be proactive in this.

To start, we want to think of the evolution of video game consoles. At one point, games consisted of 8-bit pixel characters that were moved around on a 2D level with a controller that only had one or two buttons and a direction pad. With each updated console that came out, better graphics, more controls, and ultimately a more enjoyable experience was had. But, with each upgrade came more complex challenges, harder gameplay, and a larger learning curve. Eventually, through practice and observation of the distinctions that lead to success, you adapted to the latest console and learned how to play more effectively.

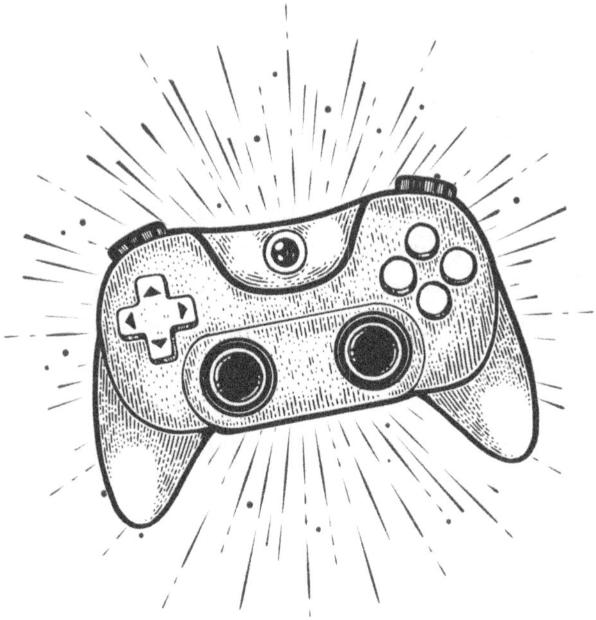

Awareness is a lot like the evolution of video game consoles. It has multiple upgrades in the form of stages. Just as with the complexity of the console and controller, your ability to dictate the character's outcomes increases with each upgrade. As you reach higher stages of awareness, you will start to spot the distinctions between things that once happened automatically without your input. Things like your emotional reactions, and missed romantic or financial opportunities you could have acted on. As you become more aware of the things that make up your life and sense of reality, you start to choose better outcomes for yourself. But just as you might find yourself overwhelmed with a new controller to a console you are unfamiliar with, awareness takes time to get used to as well.

Our mind unlocks new stages of awareness once the challenges in our life can no longer be solved by the stage we are at.

In this, your mind sheds its previously limiting awareness stage and opens up to a more complex awareness, that has the capacity to handle the life challenge you are facing. This feels a lot like looking back on your younger years with embarrassment at your certainty around something then that you know more about now.

To understand the stages, we want to imagine how we might interpret a scenario differently from each stage. Here is an example of a scenario experienced without any awareness.

Imagine you have just found out through multiple sources that your ex has started talking to one of your close friends. Your immediate reaction is jealousy as you assume that it was your ex's intention to cause you pain. Because you did not hear this from your friend, you are also filled with a feeling of distrust as you wonder how long their conversations have been going on for.

FIRST STAGE AWARENESS
SKEPTICISM

This often starts when you are able to recall a past memory of yourself wrongly interpreting a situation. When you can do this, you also understand that you are limited in your ability to know the full truth about any given circumstance. With this, you are able to step back from the once automatic emotional reaction and question if your interpretation is actually 100% true and objective. At this point, you have applied skepticism to your ability to see the whole picture, making you more mindful and hesitant about agreeing with any meaning, story, or narrative. It is an awareness that you are very unaware of, which has your mind produce thoughts along the lines of, "I know, that I do not know". This creates a gap between the stimulus of a situation and your emotional reaction to it.

Applied to the scenario:

You are able to question your assumption that your ex is trying to make you jealous and your friend is not being trustworthy. You recognize the limitations of how you know this to be true with an internal dialogue like, "I've been wrong before. I am sure there is an explanation. Plus, I have not seen anything to suggest a dynamic between them. And I have not talked to either of them about it yet." With this, you are able to hold off your impulsive emotional reaction until you find out more.

SECOND STAGE AWARENESS
CHANGE YOUR MOOD, NOT YOUR MIND

This starts as you realize that your emotional moods change your internal thoughts. You start to observe that when you are in a bad mood, you can only remember bad memories and struggle to think productively about your current circumstance. When you are in a good mood, however, you are able to remember many positive memories and also think of multiple solutions to any challenges you are currently facing. With this awareness, you notice that as your mood changes, so does your thinking about your circumstances. With this, you understand the importance of first changing your mood instead of your mind when trying to understand situations. Taking the time to only assess your challenges when you are in a good mood since you will think more productively than if you are in a bad mood. This then leads you to the realization that you should use your emotional state as a guide. Recognizing that the thoughts that show up have more to do with your mood, and less to do with your mental analysis of a situation. This stage of awareness has the mind produce thoughts like, “I know, only when I feel good" or "It is only when I feel good that I truly know".

Applied to the scenario:

You have now become aware that when you are in love with your current partner or in a new relationship, you do not care or concern yourself with your old ones. You also realize that when you are feeling good and at the top of your game, your thoughts are not concerned with the motives or intentions of your ex or close friend. You might realize that whether they are talking or not, it does not even come to mind when you are in a good mood. Therefore, you decide to just focus on being in a good mood so you don’t think about it.

THIRD STAGE AWARENESS
SELECTING MEANING

From this stage, you are fully aware that your brain makes up meaning, seeing your mind as a meaning-making machine that automatically needs to place a story to the situation. You can now control your focus to select a meaning that serves you. Realizing that this is the case, you proactively decide to interpret the story as a good one. Your thoughts at this level conclude, "I know based on what I choose".

Applied to the scenario:

You are now able to select any narrative you want about their dynamic. No longer being attached to the automatic ones. You can select the thought process of, "I feel better when I think that maybe they are just friends instead of hiding something from me. Either way, I feel better when I think what I want".

FOURTH STAGE AWARENESS
DISENGAGING FROM MEANING

This awareness comes from realizing that when you are in the process of selecting a story, neither story is true. From this, you can observe yourself existing in that space between both stories, in the gap between the situation and its potential meaning. When you are there, you come to the realization that neither the story nor your selection matter. Regardless of the meaning you assign to it, it is all still meaningless and those selections are irrelevant in the grand scheme of things. You will understand that if neither is true, then there is really no meaning to our lives. At this point, you have met yourself as the observer, seeing your mind and its meaning as completely separate from the content of your life. This can feel very detached and empty, yet freeing. The emotional conclusion of this would be a sense of knowledge that "knowing" doesn't matter.

Applied to the scenario:

Coming from this stage of awareness, you would hear the information and realize it does not matter which story or meaning you pick. You understand that regardless of your choice, their interactions are separate from you and don't matter in the overall picture of your life on earth. With that, you automatically wish them well.

FIFTH STAGE AWARENESS
ENGAGING WITH MEANING

While completely aware that it is all meaningless, you begin to ask yourself what the point of life is. At this stage, you examine the difference between selecting meaning versus not. From this, you become aware of how each of the options feels. Fully aware of the insignificance of selecting meaning, you realize that your time on this earth is most enjoyable when engaged with meaning. So from this, you willingly re-engage with meaning. But now, you do so because it is enjoyable to experience your mind doing this. So, you experience your mind creating meaning as the variety and joy of life. From this stage of awareness, you see your experience on this earth as an opportunity. You experience engagement in meaning for fun and disengage from meaning for freedom. Life becomes an experience of, "Am I in the mood for engagement or not?". If you are overwhelmed with emotion and life becomes too taxing, you disengage, stepping back from the meaning by reminding yourself of the meaninglessness of it all. But, if you are too underwhelmed and want more variety or intensity, you allow yourself to return to engaging in the meaning or story. Stepping closer to the drama of a situation and allowing your imagination to run wild with trying to make sense of it all. This understanding can be concluded as knowing for fun and not knowing for freedom.

Applied to the scenario:

You have full capacity to detach yourself from the made-up meanings of them scheming behind your back or lying about things. But with full awareness of this ability, you allow yourself to become interested for the sake of fun and enjoyment. Thinking to yourself, "I cannot wait to see this train wreck go down because I know them both and it is going to be messy. But, if it works out then that is kind of cool too. It would be interesting to see how they get along and if they are different with each other than how we were."

These five stages of awareness make up the typical journey someone goes through in becoming aware of their mind. As these are just generalized experiences, they do not need to be followed exactly. It helps to see this as a map in understanding the experience of awareness you might be feeling as you consider the contents of this book.

| A PHILOSOPHY OF ENGAGEMENT |

As a person experiences that fifth stage of awareness, they have an opportunity to operate from what we will call a philosophy of engagement. Through this, they can become aware of the different mental mechanisms that make up their thoughts. They can also disengage from the movies and meanings they create if they become too painful. Alternatively, they can also choose to relax back into these mechanisms for the sake of enjoyment, disengaging for freedom and engaging for fun. As a person does this repeatedly, they get better and more skilled at it. When this happens, a person can then experience being completely engaged in the actions of their lives. Yet, be completely free of the outcomes should those actions not work out for them. This means they can operate with a full commitment and willingness to achieve their mental movies yet be emotionally fine regardless of how those efforts turn out. It is like trying to improve your life for the sake of enjoying the act of improvement, regardless of how difficult something is. It is from this place that we make the most of our life, approaching our work, relationships, and goals as an opportunity to give it our all without concern for how that effort creates results. This is because the result was in the experience of observing ourselves maximizing the great opportunity of life.

| AN OPPORTUNITY |

While there are many approaches to your life, neither are right or wrong. You are not deficient or broken and neither is your life and the people in it. Instead, we are only ever overusing or underusing the natural mechanisms of our mind that are always available to us. With this, we turn on a light in the darkroom of our mind and reveal the imagined snakes that once limited us. Seeing our circumstance for what it is and allowing ourselves enjoyment regardless. As this book comes to a close, please take these words as an invitation to see yourself just as you are. Free of limitations with the endless possibility of what could be once you close these pages.

Made in the USA
Monee, IL
04 November 2026

67384755R00115